# Respiratory Physiology

*Raven Press Series in Physiology*

# Raven Press Series in Physiology

SERIES EDITOR

William F. Ganong, M.D.
*Professor and Chairman*
*Department of Physiology*
*University of California*
*San Francisco, California*

# Respiratory Physiology

Allan H. Mines, Ph.D.

*Associate Professor of Physiology*
*Department of Physiology*
*University of California at San Francisco*
*San Francisco, California*

Raven Press ■ New York

**Raven Press, 1140 Avenue of the Americas, New York, New York 10036**

Made in the United States of America

International Standard Book Number 0–89004–634–4
Library of Congress Catalog Card Number 80–56–58

Great care has been taken to maintain the accuracy of the information contained in the volume. However, Raven Press cannot be held responsible for errors or for any consequences arising from the use of the information contained herein.

# *Preface*

During my 18 years of teaching medical physiology to almost 5,000 students, I have tried many different instructional approaches to each subject. Some of these proved ineffective and were dropped. The techniques that I found most effective have been retained and refined, and are used in this volume. The author, and any students who may find this text helpful, are in debt to these student "guinea pigs" of mine.

What sort of book is it? No text can be all things to all students, and this one has been especially tailored for those taking a course in medical physiology. Even within this limited context, however, different sorts of coverage remain possible. The material I have selected for inclusion and the order in which I present it represents my best attempt to expedite student understanding. Reasonable teachers can (and certainly will) disagree with my choices. I apologize to them in advance.

I have also chosen to include the problems and the problem-answers following each chapter. Along with most educators, I believe that memorization of normal values and equations, and learning to understand concepts are necessary steps in a medical student's education in physiology. I do not believe students have acquired the most relevant education, however, until they can solve non-trivial problems by using the knowledge. Thus, the problems at the end of each chapter require the application of previously acquired information to new situations, some of them clinical. The answers given after the problems not only identify the correct numerical result or the correct alternative choice, but also present some of the logical sequences that might have been used in arriving at those answers.

This volume will be of interest to medical students, graduate students in physiology, and advanced students, physicians, and researchers interested in reviewing the basic physiology of the respiratory system.

Allan H. Mines

# *Acknowledgments*

I would like to thank Ms. Jeanne Ashe for preparing the manuscript. Her flying fingers and consistent attention to detail are remarkable.

My thanks go to Anne Rothman for preparing the drawings.

I am grateful to my wife, Susan, for proofreading the various stages of this text. She endured my wordiness and misspellings with equal patience.

Finally, I owe a debt to my students, on whom I have tried many of the approaches which appear in this text, as well as many others (which mercifully do not appear). I hope to repay that debt in some small way by making the study of respiratory physiology somewhat easier for students to come.

# Contents

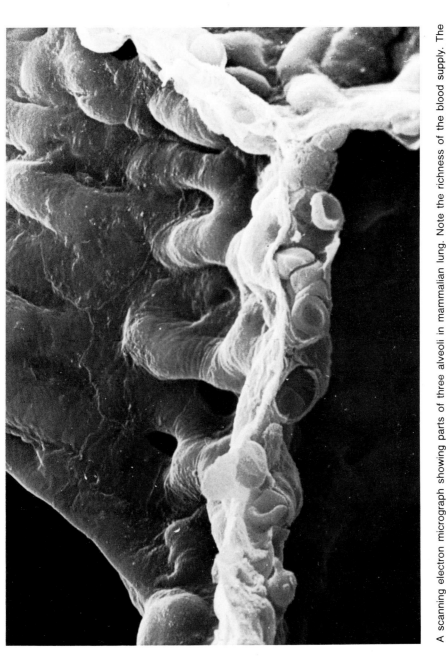

A scanning electron micrograph showing parts of three alveoli in mammalian lung. Note the richness of the blood supply. The blood vessels are packed together such that there is almost a "sheet" of blood within the alveolar septa. Note also that there is an ultra thin ($\simeq 1 \mu m$) barrier between erythrocytes and alveolar gas. Micrograph courtesy of Ewald Weibel, M. D.

# 1

# Introduction to Respiration

Respiration is often divided into two parts: Internal respiration and external respiration. The former deals with the processes by which the mitochondria metabolize various foodstuffs, usually involving $O_2$ as the oxidizing agent, and resulting in the production of high energy bonds, $CO_2$ and $H_2O$. This subject is adequately covered in any good textbook of biochemistry, and will hardly be mentioned here. The latter, external respiration, which involves the exchange of gases between the environment and the mitochondria, is the subject of this book. The first chapter is designed to give an overview of respiration: It begins with a consideration of the structure of the system from several viewpoints, and then goes into a brief description of the muscles of respiration. The symbols for variables that are commonly used in respiratory physiology are then tabulated and defined in Table 1. Next, two simple models of the respiratory system are discussed, followed by a brief consideration of the control systems that regulate our breathing. The chapter ends with the definition of the various lung volumes, and with some examples of their measurement using common methods.

## STRUCTURE

A brief consideration of the anatomy of the system is probably warranted, since an understanding of function so often depends on a knowledge of the underlying structure. The human lung is extremely complex. The main conducting tube, the trachea, divides into two bronchi, which in turn divide into two tubes each, and each of these tubes then divides into two more, and so forth. In all, there are 20–23 such divisions, resulting in 1–8 million terminal tubes. Each of these has at its end numerous blind sacs, called alveoli, where gas exchange occurs. There are about 300 million of these in man, each of which has a diameter of 75–300 $\mu$m. Breathing results in a flow of gas between the environment and the alveoli, while the right heart causes blood to flow through smaller and smaller tubes in the pulmonary circulation, and finally through a meshwork of fine capillaries encasing each alveolus, before returning to the left heart to be pumped through the body. At rest in a normal-sized person, breathing brings about 4 liters of environmental gas into the alveoli per minute

TABLE 1. *Symbols in respiratory physiology*

| General variables | | Modifying symbols | |
| --- | --- | --- | --- |
| C | Compliance | A | Alveolar gas |
| C | Concentration, content | B | Barometric |
| D | Diffusing capacity | D | Dead space gas |
| f | Respiratory frequency | E | Expired gas |
| F | Fractional concentration (dry gas) | I | Inspired gas |
| P | Gas pressure | T | Tidal gas |
| R | Resistance | | |
| R | Respiratory exchange ratio | AW | Airway |
| Q | Volume of blood | CW | Chestwall |
| Q̇ | Volume of blood per unit time | ES | Esophageal |
| V | Gas volume | IP | Intrapleural |
| V̇ | Gas volume per unit time | L | Lung |
| | | T | Total system |
| | | TC | Transchestwall |
| | | TP | Transpulmonary |
| | | TT | Transtotal system |
| | | | |
| | | a | Arterial blood |
| | | b | Blood (general) |
| | | c | Capillary blood |
| | | p | Pulmonary |
| | | t | Tissue |
| | | | |
| | | - | Mean value |
| | | · | Time derivative |

Thus, $P_{A_{O_2}}$ = Partial pressure of $O_2$ in alveolar gas
$P_{a_{O_2}}$ = Partial pressure of $O_2$ in arterial blood
$\dot{V}_{O_2}$ = $O_2$ consumption per unit time
$F_{E_{CO_2}}$ = Fraction of CO in dried, expired gas
$\dot{V}_A$ = Ventilation of the alveoli per minute or per second
$\dot{V}_A/\dot{Q}$ = Ventilation/perfusion ratio

(and about that much alveolar gas out into the environment), and the right heart pumps about 4–5.5 liters/min of blood through the pulmonary circulation. During severe exercise, the gas flow must be capable of increasing by 30- –40-fold, and the blood flow by perhaps 5- –6-fold.

These flows of gas and blood must be apportioned reasonably equitably among the 300 million alveoli. Personally, I find that numbers like million and billion, let alone the vastly larger ones which students of biology must deal with, are hard for me to comprehend. This same difficulty was expressed by a student of mine after reading this description, and we found that the concept of "1 million" became clearer to both of us when we calculated that 1 million seconds is equal to 11 days, 13 hours, and 47 minutes. A billion seconds is 31.7 years! A system designed to be able to distribute *one* fluid reasonably equitably to 300 million separate sites would be noteworthy. Our drip irrigation systems, which are now extensively employed and which must cause similar low flows of water out of each of thousands of "spigots" (some of which are elevated above the others because of nonflat terrain), are a hydraulic engineer's nightmare. The pulmonary distribution system, capable of distributing two fluids reasonably equitably among each of 300 million alveoli (some of which are above and some of which are below the pump), fair boggles the mind. In fact, although this distribution system works astonishingly well in health, the distortions of pulmonary architecture which occur pathologically can cause severe mismatching of ventilation and blood flow ($\dot{V}A/\dot{Q}$ mismatching). Under these conditions, arterialization of blood is impaired and severe disability can result.

The surface area at which these two fluids meet is very large (about 70 m²) and the average distance between the gas and blood (thickness of the membranes separating the gas and blood) is a small fraction of a micron in healthy lungs. It should be intuitively obvious to the reader that both of these factors facilitate the diffusion of gases between blood and alveolar gas. Equally obvious is that a decrease of the surface area available for exchange, or a thickening of the membranes separating the blood and gas, can lead to inadequate gas exchange, poor arterialization of blood, and clinical disability.

Even in the normal, healthy individual, about 2% of the blood draining from the body tissues bypasses the gas exchange process of the lungs. This small flow of venous blood mixes with the blood that has been arterialized in the lung, lowering the $O_2$ content of the arterial blood slightly, and lowering its partial pressure of $O_2$ quite measurably. The two circulations involved in this normal, physiological "venous admixture" are the coronary and bronchial circulations. Some of the coronary venous blood returns to the heart, not through the coronary sinus, but directly into the cavity of the left heart through the thebesian veins; some of the bronchial venous blood returns to the left heart through the pulmonary veins. Various cardiovascular and pulmonary diseases can greatly increase the magnitude of the venous admixture [also called right-to-left (R-L) shunt] causing extreme clinical disability.

On a gross anatomical scale, the lungs and airways share the chest cavity with the heart and great vessels, and the esophagus. The lungs are encased in a thin membrane called the visceral pleura, and another similar membrane, called the parietal pleura, lines the chest cavity. Between the two membranes is a very thin film of fluid that allows the two surfaces to slide past one another easily; but normally, the membranes cannot separate from one another. Why they must stay closely apposed to one another was succinctly summarized by Jere Mead in April, 1961 when he wrote in *Physiological Reviews:*

> Regard the occupancy of the chest cavity as a competition between solids, liquids, and gases. The liquids are removed down to a vestige because the capillary pressure in the visceral pleura is considerably lower than its colloid osmotic pressure. The gases are removed because the total gas pressure in venous capillary blood is considerably less than atmospheric due to the relative capacity of blood for carbon dioxide and oxygen. The lungs, chest wall, and diaphragm are then pressed into service by atmospheric pressure and occupy the space, as it were, by default.

So, normally the lungs and chest wall must move as a unit; the lung volume only changes by a liter if the chestwall volume has also changed by a liter. I emphasize this here because the diagrams we tend to make of the respiratory system often show the lungs as a smallish balloon inside a large chest cavity. We do this so that there is plenty of room to write in pressures and volumes, but the student should remember that anatomical accuracy is sacrificed in this effort.

## MUSCLES OF RESPIRATION

Normally, in quiet breathing, the inspiratory muscles pull the respiratory system above its "equilibrium volume" [Functional Residual Capacity (FRC)], then relax, allowing the elastic recoil of the system to effect expiration passively. The main inspiratory muscles are the diaphragm and the external intercostal muscles, and in quiet breathing, the diaphragm may be the only active inspiratory muscle. The diaphragm is attached all along the circumference of the lower thoracic cavity; its contraction pulls its central part down, enlarging the thoracic cavity. The motor nerves to the diaphragm leave the spinal cord in the ventral roots of C 3–5, and travel in the phrenic nerves. The external intercostal muscles are innervated by intercostal nerves, which leave the spinal cord in T 1–11. Their contraction raises the anterior end of each rib, pulling it upward and outward, and increasing the anterior–posterior diameter of the thoracic cavity. Other muscles, the "accessory" muscles of inspiration, become active only when breathing is greatly increased, as in severe muscular exercise. These include the scalenes, the sternocleidomastoids, the trapezii, and various muscles that reduce resistance to air flow. Maximal contraction of the inspiratory muscles with the glottis closed (the "Müller maneuver") can cause intrapleural pressure to become 60–100 mm Hg less than atmospheric.

Although expiration is passive during quiet breathing, it can become active when breathing is greatly increased or when significant airway obstruction exists. The abdominal muscles (including the rectus abdominus, external oblique, internal oblique, and transversus abdominus) are the principal expiratory muscles. They are innervated by nerves emerging from the spinal cord at the last six thoracic segments and at the first few lumbar ones. Their contraction increases intraabdominal pressure, thus forcing the diaphragm upward and increasing intrapleural and intrapulmonic pressures. They are absolutely essential for such functions as coughing, straining, and vomiting. The internal intercostals can also aid expiration and are innervated by intercostal nerves leaving the spinal cord at T 1–11. Forced maximal contraction of the expiratory muscles against a closed glottis (Valsalva's maneuver) can result in sustained intrapulmonary pressures above 100 mm Hg. Such pressures in the abdomen and chest will decrease venous return to the heart from the lower extremities and from the head and upper extremities. You already know that less cardiac input means less cardiac output; less cardiac output means less cerebral circulation; less cerebral circulation can mean loss of consciousness in seconds. This sequence of events leads to CNS asphyxia and unconsciousness even more rapidly if a period of hyperventilation (which constricts cerebral vessels) precedes the Valsalva maneuver.

## SYMBOLOGY

In 1951 a group of respiratory physiologists reached a consensus on a system of symbols to be used in respiratory physiology. With very few exceptions, these are used by all workers in the field today. They are internally consistent and well conceived, which makes them fairly easy to learn. They greatly simplify the consideration of the many quantitative relationships in respiratory physiology. They are listed in Table 1. We shall use these terms extensively during the respiration chapters, but I shall try always to define a symbol when it is first used.

## A MODEL OF THE RESPIRATORY SYSTEM

Let us first use these symbols to consider the simplified model of the respiratory system shown in Fig. 1. It emphasizes some things you may already know from cardiovascular physiology. The systemic and pulmonary circulations are in series with one another. During a steady state, therefore, the output of the left heart (systemic circulation) must be equal to the output of the right heart (pulmonary circulation) (ignoring, for the moment, the normal 2% R-L shunt). In the same way, the oxygen consumption ($\dot{V}_{O_2}$) that occurs at the tissues in a steady state must be exactly matched by the oxygen uptake ($\dot{V}_{O_2}$) in the lungs, and the $CO_2$ production at the tissues ($\dot{V}_{CO_2}$) must be matched by the $CO_2$ excretion by the lungs ($\dot{V}_{CO_2}$).

Arterial blood is pumped by the left heart to the tissues, where mitochondrial metabolism keeps the tissue partial pressure of $O_2$ ($Pt_{O_2}$) lower than, and the tissue partial pressure of $CO_2$ ($Pt_{CO_2}$) higher than, their respective arterial values. Thus, both gases diffuse from high partial pressure to low, resulting in $O_2$ uptake by the tissues and $CO_2$ uptake by the blood. Most tissues use nowhere near the total amount of $O_2$ present in the blood that perfuses them, and the mixed venous blood oxygen content ($C\bar{v}_{O_2}$; the bar denotes "mean value") is, at rest, normally about 75% of what it was in the arterial blood, although the partial pressure of $O_2$ in the mixed venous blood ($P\bar{v}_{O_2}$) is about 40 mm Hg, while the arterial $P_{O_2}$ ($Pa_{O_2}$) is near 100 mm Hg. This discrepancy between the fall of content and fall of partial pressure reflects the unusual sigmoid relationship between those variables in the case of $O_2$. Almost as much $CO_2$ is exchanged at the tissues as is $O_2$ [Respiratory Quotient (R.Q.) = $\dot{V}_{CO_2}/\dot{V}_{O_2}$ = about 0.8 (the dot denotes "time derivative")], yet the rise of $P_{CO_2}$ from the arterial blood to the mixed venous blood is normally only about 6–8 mm Hg. Thus, in the

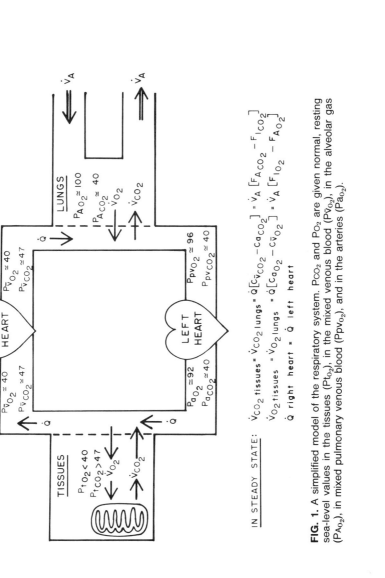

$$\text{IN STEADY STATE:} \quad \dot{V}_{CO_2 \, tissues} = \dot{V}_{CO_2 \, lungs} = \dot{Q}\left[C_{\bar{v}_{CO_2}} - Ca_{CO_2}\right] = \dot{V}_A \left[F_{A_{CO_2}} - F_{I_{CO_2}}\right]$$

$$\dot{V}_{O_2 \, tissues} = \dot{V}_{O_2 \, lungs} = \dot{Q}\left[Ca_{O_2} - C\bar{v}_{O_2}\right] = \dot{V}_A \left[F_{I_{O_2}} - F_{A_{O_2}}\right]$$

$$\dot{Q} \text{ right heart} = \dot{Q} \text{ left heart}$$

**FIG. 1.** A simplified model of the respiratory system. $P_{CO_2}$ and $P_{O_2}$ are given normal, resting sea-level values in the tissues ($Pt_{O_2}$), in the mixed venous blood ($P\bar{v}_{O_2}$), in the alveolar gas ($PA_{O_2}$), in mixed pulmonary venous blood ($Ppv_{O_2}$), and in the arteries ($Pa_{O_2}$).

normal range the curve relating content of $CO_2$ to its partial pressure has a very different shape from that of the $O_2$ curve.

The mixed venous blood is then pumped by the right heart to the lungs where it exchanges with alveolar gas, losing $CO_2$ to the gas and gaining $O_2$ from it. The partial pressures in the mixed pulmonary venous blood are normally very nearly the same as those in mixed alveolar gas, and the partial pressures and contents in arterial blood are again very nearly the same as those in mixed pulmonary venous blood. The alveolar ventilation ($\dot{V}A$) brings a flow of fresh environmental gas, which is rich in $O_2$ (20.93%) and almost free of $CO_2$ (0.04%), through the alveoli. This flow of gas tends to replace the $O_2$ taken up by the blood and to carry the $CO_2$ given off by the blood out into the environment. Again in the steady state, the amounts of $O_2$ and $CO_2$ exchanged at the alveolar membranes must be equal to the amounts exchanged with environment per minute.

## PRESSURE PROFILE OF $O_2$ FROM ENVIRONMENT TO MITOCHONDRION

The respiratory system can also be viewed as a delivery system that passes $O_2$ down a series of steps between environment and mitochondrion, as seen in Fig. 2. There is a limited "pressure head" for that delivery, which is set by $Po_2$ in the environmental gas, which in turn is determined by the barometric pressure times the fraction of the dry gas molecules which are $O_2$ ($PB \times Fo_2$). If the environmental gas is totally dry, which normally occurs only if a subject breathes from a tank of dried compressed air, then the environmental $Po_2 = 760 \times 0.2093 = 159$ mm Hg. It is easy to see that lowering either $PB$ (as in the ascent to high altitude) or $Fo_2$ (as in breathing a mixture of air and $N_2$) will lower the available "pressure head" for $O_2$ delivery, and tend to lower the maximum possible $\dot{V}o_2$. As soon as the gas enters the warm, moist respiratory tract it is humidified, and by the time it reaches the trachea it has become saturated with water vapor. At a body temperature of 37°C, the water vapor pressure is 47 mm Hg, and the total pressure exerted by the other gases ($O_2$, $N_2$, $CO_2$, etc.) can then be only $760 - 47 = 713$ mm Hg. The $Po_2$ in the trachea, defined as the inspired $Po_2$ ($PI_{o_2}$), is then ($PB - PH_2O$) ($FI_{o_2}$) = 713 mm Hg (0.2093) = 149 mm Hg. So, $Po_2$ decreased as the gas became humidified, simply because the water vapor diluted the $O_2$. The gas then passes into the alveoli where its $Po_2$ (the $PA_{o_2}$) is determined by a balance of two processes. The alveolar ventilation ($\dot{V}A$) brings a flow of $O_2$-rich gas into the alveoli and tends to raise $PA_{o_2}$, while the pulmonary blood flow ($\dot{Q}$) removes $O_2$ from the alveolar gas and tends to lower $PA_{o_2}$. As $\dot{V}A$ increases, clearly $PA_{o_2}$ will tend to be brought closer to $PI_{o_2}$, and vice versa. In this case, $PA_{o_2}$ is shown to be a nice, normal sea-level value of 100 mm Hg. The pulmonary venous blood, here shown to have a $Po_2$ of 96 mm Hg, normally has a slightly lower $Po_2$ than the mixed alveolar gas. The two possible contributors to this drop of

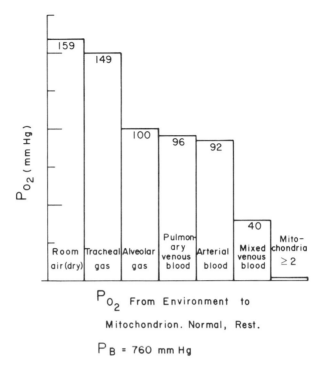

**FIG. 2.** Oxygen pressure profile from environment to mitochondrion in a normal resting male at sea level.

$Po_2$ are $\dot{V}A/\dot{Q}$ mismatching and diffusion difficulties, but normally at sea level the latter contribution is too small to measure. As already mentioned in this chapter, however, pulmonary disease can result in either of these factors producing a drop in $Po_2$, which can be severely debilitating. By the time the arterialized blood from the lungs has mixed with the 2% R-L shunt (coronary and bronchial circulations), and has been pumped into the systemic arteries, its $Po_2$ (now the arterial $Po_2$ or $Pa_{o_2}$) has decreased still further, and is here shown to be 92 mm Hg. This small difference of 8 mm Hg between $PA_{o_2}$ and $Pa_{o_2}$ can obviously be increased greatly if the R-L shunt is larger.

Since the arterial walls are far too thick to allow any significant gas exchange, neither $Pa_{o_2}$ nor the $O_2$ content changes until the blood reaches the capillaries, where only a single endothelial cell separates blood from tissue. Tissue $Po_2$ ($Pt_{o_2}$) is kept quite low ($< 40$ mm Hg) so that $O_2$ diffuses from blood to tissue rapidly near the arterial end of the capillary, where the difference in $Po_2$ is large ($92 - Pt_{o_2}$), and then less and less rapidly as the $Po_2$ in the capillary decreases. The $O_2$, still following its partial pressure gradient, diffuses through the extracellular fluid, into the cells, finally to reach the mitochondria, the lowest level in this $O_2$ transport cascade, where $Po_2$ may get as low as 1–3 mm Hg. Here, $O_2$ is used to oxidize $H_2$ and C, which is the ultimate purpose of this $O_2$ delivery system. The blood, having passed through the tissue capillaries, now returns to the right heart through the systemic veins, its $P_{O_2}$ having been decreased to about 40 mm Hg.

## CONTROL OF RESPIRATORY SYSTEM

Unlike the heart, which has its own intrinsic rhythm, the respiratory muscles do not "beat" on their own, and therefore respiration needs to have neural systems capable of generating and maintaining a regular breathing cycle to carry out gas exchange between environment and alveoli. We know that the organism's environment is subject to change (ascent to high altitude, scuba diving, etc.) and that mitochondrial activity is subject to change (muscular exercise, body temperature change, altered thyroid function, etc.). Thus, there is clearly a need for systems that will modify this basic regular breathing cycle by achieving rates of gas exchange that will satisfy bodily needs under a wide variety of functional states. These systems must have receptors to sample the parameters of importance to the respiratory system ($P_{O_2}$, $P_{CO_2}$, pH, state of lung inflation, level of muscular activity, etc.). Using that information, and setting priorities when conflicting needs exist, the systems must drive the muscles of respiration smoothly, dependably, and automatically. They must be capable of voluntary override to allow for speech and the myriad other activities in which we engage using nose and mouth. These systems will be discussed at some length in the chapter entitled "Regulation of Breathing."

## LUNG VOLUMES

Clinically, it is useful to be able to measure the volume of gas in the lungs under a number of different circumstances. The various divisions and subdivisions of the lung volume are shown in Fig. 3. Total Lung Capacity (TLC) is the maximum amount of gas the lung can contain *in vivo*, when the subject inspires as much as he can. When the subject starts from that position of maximum inflation, and expires as much gas as he can, he is exhaling his Vital Capacity (VC). At this point, there will be a significant amount of gas still left in the lung, the Residual Volume (RV), which cannot be exhaled *in vivo*. Normally, however, people do not exhale down to RV with each breath. During quiet breathing, they exhale down to FRC, at which point the elastic recoils of the two components (lungs and chest wall) just balance one another. FRC, then, is the volume to which the respiratory system returns at the end of a normal quiet breath, and is about 40% of the TLC. If a subject inhales as much as he can, beginning at FRC, he inhales his Inspiratory Capacity (IC). Normally, however, people inhale much smaller volumes with each quiet breath, called Tidal Volumes ($V_T$). After having inhaled a tidal volume, a person still has a considerable Inspiratory Reserve Volume (IRV) between end-inspiration and

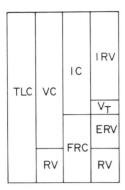

**FIG. 3.** Lung volumes in a healthy young male.

TLC. After having exhaled normally down to FRC, a person has a smaller, but still considerable, Expiratory Reserve Volume (ERV) between FRC and RV.

## MEASUREMENT OF LUNG VOLUMES

It is easy to measure those lung volumes not involving the RV with a simple spirometer, shown in Fig. 4. It is simply an upside-down water-sealed can (called a bell) whose movements are recorded on moving paper. When a subject is made to breathe into and out of the spirometer, his breathing movements are traced on the paper. If, for instance, beginning at TLC, he exhales down to

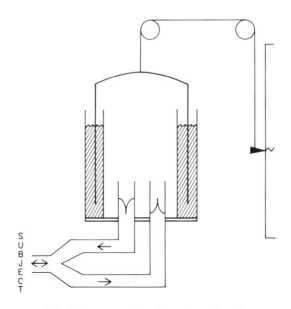

**FIG. 4.** A cross section through a spirometer.

RV, the pen will have moved a vertical distance proportional to his VC. All one needs to know is the constant of proportionality (which turns out to be the cross-sectional area of the bell) to calculate the volume that has been put into the bell (the volume of the right-circular cylinder which has been filled) as the subject exhaled his VC. Of course, the gas in the lungs was at 37°C and saturated with $H_2O$ at that temperature (Body Temperature and Pressure, Saturated, or BTPS), while the gas will have decreased in volume as it entered the spirometer, which is at Ambient Temperature and Pressure, Saturated, or ATPS, so an ideal gas correction is necessary. Assuming that $P_B = 760$ mm Hg, body temperature $= 37°C$ (at which temperature the vapor pressure of $H_2O$ is 47 mm Hg), and spirometer temperature $= 25°C$ (at which temperature $P_{H_2O} = 24$ mm Hg), the calculation proceeds as follows:

$$\frac{P_1V_1}{T_1} = \frac{P_2V_2}{T_2}$$
$$V_2 = \frac{P_1V_1T_2}{T_1P_2} = \frac{(736 \text{ mm Hg})(V_1)(310°K)}{(298°K)(713 \text{ mm Hg})}$$

Thus, $V_2 = 1.074(V_1)$, or, the actual volume moved out of the lungs is 7.4% greater than the volume moved into the spirometer. In a similar fashion, one could measure IC, IRV, ERV, and $V_T$, but wouldn't know the value of TLC, RV, or FRC without more information.

The additional information can be gotten through the use of either a volume of dilution method or a Boyle's law method. You may already have become familiar with the principle behind the volumes of dilution method. Figure 5 shows one way that it can be used to measure FRC, called the helium closed circuit method. At FRC, a subject begins rebreathing from a bag that initially contains 2 liters of 10% He. He continues to rebreathe until mixing is complete and the concentration of He is the same in the bag and the lungs. Since negligible amounts of He are taken up by the body, the initial amount of He present only in the bag must equal the final amount of He "present in bag and lungs." The calculation proceeds as follows:

$$\text{Initial amount of He} = \text{Final amount of He}$$
$$V_L(\%He)_i + V_{bag}(\%He)_i = (V_L + V_{bag})(\%He)_f$$
$$0 + 2 \text{ liters }(0.1) = (V_L + 2 \text{ liters})(0.05)$$
$$0.2 \text{ liters} = 0.05V_L + 0.1 \text{ liter}$$
$$2 \text{ liters} = V_L$$

where $V_L$ and $V_{bag}$ are the volumes of lung and bag, respectively, and i and f refer to the initial and final (complete mixing) situations. This type of method will measure the volume of all gas able to exchange with the bag He, but will not measure that which is trapped beyond occluded airways.

The Boyle's law method measures the total Thoracic Gas Volume (TGV), whether in free communication with the airways or not. Boyle's law simply

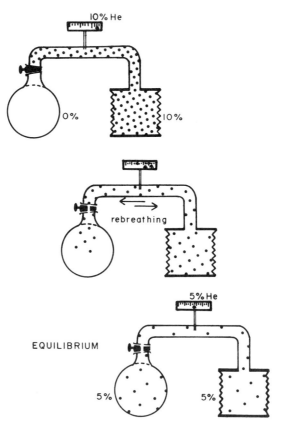

**FIG. 5.** Measurement of FRC: Helium closed-circuit technique. (Reproduced with permission from Comroe, J. H., Jr., et al.: *The Lung: Clinical Physiology and Pulmonary Function Tests,* 2nd Ed. Copyright © 1962 by Year Book Medical Publishers, Chicago.)

states that the pressure times the volume of a gas is constant, provided that both the number of moles and the temperature stay constant, or $P_1V_1 = P_2V_2$. This method requires the use of a body plethysmograph, one type of which is shown in Fig. 6. The subject is seated within an airtight box, breathing the outside air through a tube. A pressure gauge samples the pressure in the tube near his mouth, which will be equal to alveolar pressure only if there is no flow of gas through the tube. The volume changes of his lung are measured accurately by the Krogh spirometer. As he breathes in, expanding his chest by 1 liter, 1 liter of air around him is displaced up into the Krogh spirometer, and vice versa. To measure the FRC, one simply occludes the airway when the subject has just completed a normal expiration (subject at FRC) by turning the stopcock 90° counterclockwise. The subject makes inspiratory and expiratory efforts against the closed airway, thus decompressing and compressing the gas in his lungs, and these volume changes continue to be recorded by the Krogh

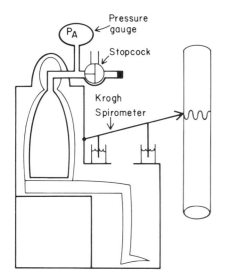

**FIG. 6.** The "Mead-type" body plethysmograph. The subject breathes normally while the stopcock is connected to the environment. Then the stopcock is turned to occlude the airway while the subject makes inspiratory and expiratory efforts, his alveolar pressure being recorded using a pressure gauge connected to the airway proximal to the stopcock. The Krogh spirometer measures $\Delta V$, and thus one determines $\Delta V/\Delta P$, and can calculate TGV.

spirometer. Since the airway is occluded (no gas flow), the pressure gauge measures the changes in pressure of the lung gas associated with these volume changes. Assuming that the change in volume $(\Delta V) = 71$ ml, and that the change in lung gas pressure $(\Delta P) = 20$ mm Hg, and that $P_B = 760$ mm Hg, the calculation proceeds as follows:

$$PV = (P + \Delta P)(V - \Delta V)$$

Multiplying out

$$PV = PV - P\Delta V + V\Delta P - \Delta P\Delta V$$

Adding out PV's, rearranging, and factoring

$$V = \frac{\Delta V\,(P + \Delta P)}{\Delta P}$$

Since $\Delta P$ is quite small relative to P (20 mm Hg versus 713 mm Hg), then

$$V = \frac{\Delta V}{\Delta P}\,(P)$$

$$V = \frac{71 \text{ ml }(713 \text{ mm Hg})}{20 \text{ mm Hg}} = 2{,}538 \text{ ml} = \text{TGV at FRC}$$

The P used is $P_B - P_{H_2O}$ because $P_{H_2O}$ remains constant during the volume and pressure changes involved in this measurement, some $H_2O$ evaporating from lung surfaces during inspiratory attempts, and some condensing during expiratory attempts. Only the other, dry gases, are obeying Boyle's law.

In health, the values obtained for RV, TLC, and FRC by the volumes of dilution method should equal the values obtained by the Boyle's law method.

However, respiratory disease, which causes some areas of the lung to be temporarily nonventilated (emphysema, for instance), can cause significant differences in the measurements obtained by the two different methods. Emphysema may also cause FRC, RV, and TLC to be larger than normal (the so-called "barrel chest") due to loss of lung elastic recoil. The elastic recoil of lungs and chestwall, as well as the interaction between these two organs, will be considered in some detail in the next chapter.

## REFERENCES

1. Agostoni, E. (1964): Action of respiratory muscles. In: *Handbook of Physiology, Sect. 3: Respiration,* edited by W. O. Fenn and H. Rahn, Vol. 1, p. 377. American Physiological Society, Washington, D.C.
2. Comroe, J. H., Jr. (1962): *The Lung.* Year Book Medical Publishers, Chicago.
3. Krahl, V. E. (1964): Anatomy of the mammalian lung. In: *Handbook of Physiology, Sect. 3: Respiration,* edited by W. O. Fenn and H. Rahn, Vol. 1, p. 213. American Physiological Society, Washington, D.C.
4. Pappenheimer, J. R. (1950): Standardization of definitions and symbols in respiratory physiology. *Fed. Proc.,* 9:602–605.
5. Weibel, E. R. (1964): Morphometrics of the lung. In: *Handbook of Physiology, Sect. 3: Respiration,* edited by W. O. Fenn and H. Rahn, Vol. 1, p. 285. American Physiological Society, Washington, D.C.

## PROBLEMS

1. Between successive steps along the $O_2$ transport pathway, the $Po_2$ drops. Thus, it is about 150 mm Hg in the inspired gas, only about 100 mm Hg in the alveoli normally, etc. Below is a list of some of these steps along the $O_2$ transport pathway, and the normal, sea-level resting values of $Po_2$ that might be found there (in parentheses). Also listed below are six conditions that would cause $Po_2$ to drop more than it normally does between two successive steps. For each condition (1–6), select a letter identifying the pair of steps between which the drop in $Po_2$ would be increased most by the condition stated.

Conditions

1. Heavy exercise (running)
2. Hypoventilation
3. Breathing air at high altitude (resting)
4. Worsening of $\dot{V}A/\dot{Q}$ matching
5. Abnormally thickened alveolar membranes

Steps along $O_2$ transport pathway

A. $\left\{\begin{array}{l}\text{Inspired gas in trachea (150 mm Hg)}\end{array}\right.$

B. $\left\{\begin{array}{l}\text{Mean alveolar gas (100 mm Hg)}\end{array}\right.$

C. $\left\{\begin{array}{l}\text{Mixed pulmonary venous blood (95 mm Hg)}\end{array}\right.$

D. $\left\{\begin{array}{l}\text{Aortic blood (90 mm Hg)}\end{array}\right.$

E. $\left\{\begin{array}{l}\text{Inferior vena caval blood (40 mm Hg)}\\ \text{Pulmonary arterial blood (40 mm Hg)}\end{array}\right.$

6. Increased R-L shunting via the coronary circulation

F. {None of the above satisfies the condition

2. A child is connected, at FRC, to a bag containing 2 liters of 8% He, 92% $O_2$. He rebreathes from the bag until mixing is complete, at which time the He concentration in the bag is 4.6%. What is the value of the child's FRC?

3. A patient suffers a severed spinal cord in an automobile accident. He is still able to breathe fairly well, but finds that he is unable to forcibly exhale, as in blowing out a match. He is paralyzed from the neck down.

   A. Localize the level at which the spinal cord is severed as well as you can from this information.
   B. What problems of a respiratory nature is this patient likely to experience?

4. Given the following data obtained from a healthy child breathing normal room air in a steady state:

$P_B = 637$ mm Hg
Body temp. $= 37°C$
$\dot{V}_A$, STPD $= 2.0$ liters/min
$\dot{V}_{CO_2} = 100$ ml/min, STPD
$\dot{V}_{O_2} = 125$ ml/min, STPD
$P_{A_{O_2}} = 84.4$ mm Hg

Calculate
A. $F_{A_{O_2}}$
B. $P_{I_{O_2}}$
C. R.Q.
D. $\dot{V}_A$, BTPS

## ANSWERS

1. *Condition 1:* Heavy exercise (running) will cause much more $O_2$ to be removed from the blood perfusing the lower limbs, lowering its $P_{O_2}$ dramatically. This abnormally low $P_{O_2}$ will be seen in the blood in the inferior vena cava. Thus, the answer is step D.

   *Condition 2:* Hypoventilation will cause less $O_2$-rich fresh gas to be brought into the alveoli each minute, and continued uptake by the blood will lower alveolar $P_{O_2}$. Thus, the answer is step A.

   *Condition 3:* Air at high altitude will have a lower $P_B$, and therefore a lower $P_{I_{O_2}}$. The unusual drop in $P_{O_2}$ therefore occurs in the inspired gas in the trachea, and not between any two successive steps. Thus, the answer is step F.

*Condition 4:* As $\dot{V}A/\dot{Q}$ matching worsens, the drop in $P_{O_2}$ between alveolar gas and mixed pulmonary venous blood will increase. Thus, the answer is step **B**.

*Condition 5:* Abnormally thickened alveolar membranes will likewise cause a larger than normal drop in the $P_{O_2}$ between alveolar gas and mixed pulmonary venous blood. Thus, the answer is step **B**.

*Condition 6:* Increased R-L shunting via the coronary circulation will add more than the usual amounts of venous blood to the plumonary venous blood as it enters the left side of the heart, resulting in a greater than normal drop in $P_{O_2}$ between mixed pulmonary venous blood and blood in the aorta. Thus, the answer is step **C**.

2.
$$Vbag\,(FHe) = (Vbag + VL)\,(FHe)_f$$
$$VL = \frac{Vbag\,(FHe)_i - Vbag\,(FHe)_f}{(FHe)_f} = 1.48 \text{ liters at FRC}$$

where $VL$ and $Vbag$ are the volumes of lung and bag, respectively, and i and f refer to the initial and final situations.

3. **A:** Since the patient cannot forcibly exhale, his expiratory muscles are paralyzed. These are innervated by nerves leaving the spinal cord in the thoracic and lumbar regions. This information, plus his paralysis from the neck down puts the lesion in the cervical region. Since he can breathe fairly well, his diaphragm is innervated normally, and thus the lesion must be at C6-C7. **B:** Coughing is impossible without the expiratory muscles, and coughing helps maintain airways hygiene. Thus, this individual will be more at risk than a normal person as regards infectious diseases of the lungs and airways.

4. **A:** $FA_{O_2}$ is simply $PA_{O_2}/(PB - PH_2O) = 84.4/591 = 0.14$.
   **B:** $PI_{O_2}$ is $(PB - PH_2O)\,(FI_{O_2})$, and since the child is breathing normal room air, whose $FI_{O_2}$ is 0.2093, the answer is 123.7 mm Hg.
   **C:** The R.Q. is simply $\dot{V}CO_2/\dot{V}O_2 = 100/125 = 0.80$.
   **D:** To convert from STPD to BTPS, one uses the ideal gas laws, making corrections for both temperature and pressure:

$$\frac{PV}{T} = \frac{P_1 V_1}{T_1}$$

$$V_1 = \frac{PVT_1}{P_1 T} = \frac{760 \text{ mm Hg (2 liters/min, STPD) } (310^\circ K)}{(273^\circ K)\,(591 \text{ mm Hg})}$$

$$= 2.92 \text{ liters/min, BTPS}$$

# 2

# *Mechanics of Breathing*

Periodic inflation and deflation of the lungs maintains a flow of environmental gas through the alveoli. To bring about this flow, the respiratory muscles must do work both to stretch the elastic components of the respiratory system and to overcome resistance to flow. During quiet breathing, the muscles are able to accomplish this work while using only about one-tenth of one percent of the total body $O_2$ consumption. These muscles and their innervations are described in Chapter 1.

For the student to acquire a thorough understanding of this subject, which is the goal of this chapter, he must characterize the behavior of the system in well-defined physical terms. The chapter thus begins with a consideration of pressures, pressure units, and differential pressures. It then proceeds to a definition of compliance (distensibility), and a consideration of the compliances of the lungs alone, chestwall alone, and lungs and chestwall when linked together. Surface tension, which accounts for much of the elastic recoil of the lung, is next considered in some detail. The chapter then proceeds to discuss resistances to flow; what normally keeps them comfortably low, and how lung disease can cause them to become cripplingly high. As usual, there are problems to work at the end of the chapter, which allow the student to evaluate whether he or she understands the material well enough to use it effectively.

## PRESSURES

Pressure in a liquid or gas is exerted equally in every direction. When the fluid under pressure meets a solid boundary, the pressure exerts a force on the boundary. If the boundary is flat, the force exerted on it is equal to pressure times area: $F = P \times A$. If the boundary is curved, some form of LaPlace's law applies in which tension is proportional to pressure times radius of curvature: $T \propto P \times R$.

You may have been introduced to units of pressure in cardiovascular physiology. Respiratory physiologists have frequently found centimeters of water (cm $H_2O$) to be the most convenient measuring unit because the pressures they deal with are usually fairly low. It is a smaller unit than millimeters of mercury (mm Hg), each centimeter of water being about 74% of a millimeter of mercury (1 atm = 760 mm Hg = 1,033 cm $H_2O$). In centimeter-gram-second (cgs) units, which must be used when dealing with surface tension, 1 cm $H_2O$ = 980 dynes/cm². In meter-kilogram-second (mks) units, 1 cm $H_2O$ = 98 Newtons/ m²; 1 atm ≃ 10⁵ N/m². Or, according to yet another system of pressure units, 1 N/m² ≅ 0.01 cm $H_2O$ = 1 Pascal. Thus, 1,000 N/M² = kPa ≅ 10 cm $H_2O$ ≅ 7 mm Hg. These many units are mentioned without any strong preference being put forward by the author because the student will probably see all of them at one time or another in his or her career. Since most of the published data uses centimeters of water as the unit, I shall use that unit preferentially in this chapter.

When a pressure is measured and found to be, for instance, 10 cm $H_2O$, the next question must be, "relative to what?" If no further information is given, physiologists assume that the pressure was measured *relative to atmospheric pressure*. For instance, a normal mean arterial blood pressure is about 95 mm Hg *greater* than atmospheric pressure. If the measurement were made at sea level, where the barometric pressure (PB) equals 760 mm Hg, the absolute blood pressure (relative to a vacuum) would be 855 mm Hg.

When one deals with hollow organs, however, as physiologists must, one not only makes measurements of pressures relative to atmospheric pressure but also calculates or measures pressure differences across walls of those organs, called transmural ("across-the-wall") pressures. You may have already considered these transmural pressures as they related to blood vessels and the heart chambers. Figure 1 shows that transmural pressures (PTM) must be measured across spherical structures such as a balloon, an alveolus, or a lung, for it is the PTM which is the distending pressure in each case. PTM is always defined as $P_{in} - P_{out}$.

The mammalian respiratory system, even when considered simplistically as two balloons (lungs and chestwall) one inside the other as in Fig. 2, becomes quite complex. Firstly, to quantitate the elastic characteristics of the lungs, PTM must be determined across the lung (called the transpulmonary pressure or PTP) by subtracting the intrapleural pressure from the alveolar pressure

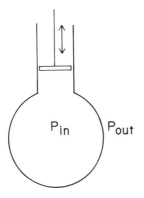

**FIG. 1.** The transmural pressure of an organ like the lung is defined as the pressure inside the organ minus the pressure outside it; PTM = $P_{in} - P_{out}$.

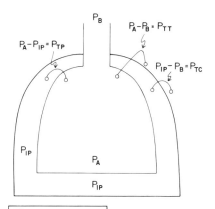

$P_B$

$P_A - P_{IP} = P_{TP}$

$P_A - P_B = P_{TT}$

$P_{IP} - P_B = P_{TC}$

$P_{IP}$

$P_A$

$P_{IP}$

**FIG. 2.** There are three transmural pressures to consider in the respiratory system. (a) $P_{TP}$ = $P_A$ − $P_{IP}$; (b) $P_{TC}$ = $P_{IP}$ − $P_B$; and (c) $P_{TT}$ = $P_A$ − $P_B$. $P_A$, alveolar pressure; $P_{IP}$, intrapleural pressure; $P_B$, barometric pressure; $P_{TP}$, transpulmonary pressure; $P_{TC}$, transchestwall pressure; $P_{TT}$, transtotal system pressure.

TP= transpulmonary
TC= trans chest wall
TT= trans total system

($P_A$ − $P_{IP}$). This measurement must be made at each of a series of volumes, and, if drops in pressure due to flow resistance are to be absent, measurement must also be made during conditions of no flow. Similarly, to quantitate the elastic characteristics of the chestwall, the transmural pressure across the chestwall ($P_{TC}$ = $P_{IP}$ − $P_B$) must be measured at each of a series of volumes during no flow. Further, since breathing normally occurs by virtue of the contractions of muscles in the chestwall, one must insure that the muscles are relaxed if one wishes to define the *passive* elastic characteristics of the chestwall. In this sense the lungs are easier to deal with than the chestwall, for their movements are always brought about by "extrinsic" forces such as respiratory muscles or respiratory pumps.

## COMPLIANCE AND ELASTANCE

When physicists wish to quantitate the elastic characteristics of a structure, they measure its elastance, or the reciprocal of that, its compliance. The best common synonym for elastance is probably stiffness, and that for compliance is probably distensibility. The words elasticity and elastic are to be avoided since their meanings are so unclear. To say that a structure is elastic means to most of us that it stretches easily; to a physicist that statement means that the energy expended in distorting the structure is largely recovered as it recoils. The terms elastance and compliance are less ambiguous. Thus, a tennis ball has less elastance than a superball, which has less elastance than a steel ball, which has less elastance than a glass ball. The tennis ball has high compliance, being easily distended; it has low elastance, however.

Compliance is far more commonly measured than is elastance in respiratory physiology, and I would thus like to discuss it from now on. Compliance (C) is equal to a change in dimensions divided by a change in the force, tension,

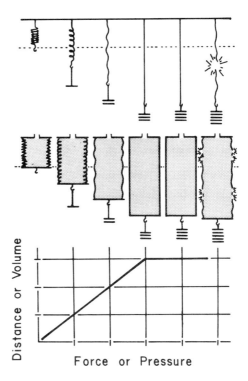

**FIG. 3.** Hooke's law applied to a spring and to the lungs. For an elastic structure, the increase in length (or volume) varies directly with the increase in force (or pressure) until the elastic limit is reached. This linear relationship applies equally to normal lungs, over the physiological range. (Reproduced with permission from Comroe, J. H., Jr., et al.: *The Lung: Clinical Physiology and Pulmonary Function Tests,* 2nd Ed. Copyright © 1962 by Year Book Medical Publishers, Chicago.)

or pressure applied (or strain/stress). Here strain refers to the dimensional change, and stress refers to the agency producing that change. Robert Hooke, in the late 1600's, found that the ratio of strain/stress was constant for an elastic structure until the elastic limit was reached. Hooke's law, as applied to a spring and to a lung-like structure, is illustrated in Fig. 3. It shows that the increase in length or volume of an elastic structure varies directly with the increase in force or pressure applied to it until an elastic limit is reached. Many physiological structures obey this linear relationship over at least a part of their range of movement.

## VOLUME VERSUS PRESSURE CURVE OF LUNGS AND CHESTWALL—STATIC (NO FLOW)

It is easy to measure the volume versus pressure curve of lungs removed at autopsy because one can easily measure the transmural pressure across the lungs. One simply determines the pressure inside the lungs, the alveolar pressure (PA), and subtracts the pressure outside the lungs from it, the barometric pressure (PB), to derive the transpulmonary pressure (PTP) at each of a series of lung volumes during conditions of no flow. In order to begin the determination at zero volume, one would have to de-gas the lungs (by subjecting them to a vacuum) since there are a few hundred milliliters of gas trapped in normal human lungs when they are removed from the chest cavity and allowed to reach their "rest" or "equilibrium" volume. The lungs can also approach their "rest" or "equilibrium" volume when the chest is opened at surgery, when a patient suffers penetrating wounds of the chestwall, or when a part of the lung ruptures. This situation, in which air is allowed to enter the intrapleural space, is called, quite reasonably, pneumothorax. Breathing can be painful, difficult, or impossible depending on the magnitude and location of the pneumothorax.

In a normal, healthy individual, of course, there is no air in the intrapleural space, and the lung volume never drops below residual volume (considerably greater than the "rest" or "equilibrium" volume). In such a normal individual, one can still determine the volume/pressure curve of the lungs *in vivo*. The same parameters must be measured: Volume of the lungs (V), the pressure within the lungs, the alveolar pressure (PA), and that immediately outside the lungs, the intrapleural pressure (PIP), during each of a series of briefly maintained volumes. The volume changes of the lungs can be measured easily with a simple spirometer, and PA can be measured by measuring airway pressure when it is equal to PA (conditions of no flow). Measuring PIP is more of a problem. It is possible to insert a needle into the potential intrapleural space, inject a few hundred milliliters of sterile air to convert the potential space into a real one, and use the pressure of the gas in this space as a measure of the PIP. The procedure is uncomfortable and risky and thus seldom used.

The use of an esophageal balloon offers an attractive alternative (see Fig. 4). A fine tube whose open end is covered by a very thin-walled flaccid balloon is passed, via the nose, into the lower third of the esophagus. The esophagus shares the pleural space with the lungs and heart, and is itself very flaccid except when swallowing. Since its walls are so loose, no difference in pressure develops between its inside and its outside (PIP), and changes in intraesophageal pressure (PES) mimic very closely changes in PIP. Likewise, since very little air is put into the balloon, its walls stay very flaccid, and no difference in pressure develops between balloon pressure and PES. Thus, changes in balloon pressure, which can be measured, are identical to changes in PIP, as closely as we can tell.[1] The esophageal balloon technique gives an accurate determination of *changes* in PIP, rather than *the* PIP primarily because PIP varies according to where it is measured, becoming more subatmospheric as one approaches

---

[1] The student may enjoy proving, using LaPlace's law for cylinders, that the pressure within a properly used esophageal balloon reflects accurately the pressure just outside the esophagus at that level.

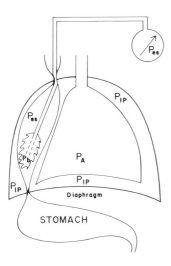

**FIG. 4.** Esophageal pressure (Pes) can be used as a good measure of intrapleural pressure (Pip) if the esophageal walls are flaccid. Balloon pressure ($P_b$) accurately reflects Pes if the walls of the balloon are flaccid.

the lung apices in the upright position. The actual PES at any given moment is apparently some average of the PIP's at the various levels of the pleural space.

Let us now consider a normal person lying at rest, between breaths. His lung volume is at functional residual capacity (FRC), the relaxation volume of the whole respiratory system. Intrapleural pressure is subatmospheric. Thus, the lungs are being held inflated at a volume greater than their equilibrium volume (PTP is greater than zero), and the chestwall is being held "crushed down" to a volume less than its equilibrium volume (PTC is less than zero or negative). Viewed slightly differently, the reason the system stays balanced at FRC is because the tendency of the lungs to get smaller is exactly counteracted by the tendency of the chestwall to get larger. If PIP were allowed to become equal to atmospheric through a hole in the chestwall, the lungs would collapse as the chestwall expanded. Let us consider the same person still lying at rest, but now with his muscles completely paralyzed so that both lungs and chestwall behave passively. Using a mechanical respirator, we can inflate the whole system to total lung capacity (TLC), then deflate it in successive increments of a liter or half a liter until residual volume (RV) is reached. Measuring PA, PIP, and PB allows us to calculate the transpulmonary pressure (PTP), the transchestwall pressure (PTC), and the transtotal system pressure (PTT) during the deflation. The data that one might get in a healthy person of normal size are listed in Table 1 and graphed in Fig. 5. In Fig. 5, the curve marked "L" is the lung curve (V versus PTP), the curve marked "CW" is the chestwall curve (V versus PTC), and the curve marked "T" is the total system curve (V versus PTT). Since compliance (C) = the change in volume divided by the change in transmural pressure ($\Delta V/\Delta PTM$), the slope at any point of any of these curves is the compliance at that point in the curve.

TABLE 1. *Mechanical factors in breathing*

| | | | | | Sample data from inflating the lungs of a completely paralyzed person | | | | |
| | A | B | C | D | E | F | G | H | I |
| | Vol. of gas in lungs (liters) | $P_A$ (cm $H_2O$) | | ←Difference→ $P_{TP}$ | | $P_{ES}$ (cm $H_2O$) | ←Difference→ $P_{TC}$ | | Pressure outside of chest (cm $H_2O$) |
| | | | $C_T$ | | $C_L$ | | | | $C_{CW}$ |
| TLC | 6.0 | 43 | | ←30→ | 0.06 | 13 | ←13→ | 0.17 | 0 = $P_B$ |
| | 5.5 | 31 | 0.04 | ←21→ | 0.17 | 10 | ←10→ | 0.20 | 0 |
| | 4.5 | 20 | 0.09 | ←15→ | 0.20 | 5 | ← 5→ | 0.20 | 0 |
| | 3.5 | 10 | 0.10 | ←10→ | 0.20 | 0 | ↓ 0→ | 0.20 | 0 |
| FRC | 2.5 | 0 | 0.10 | ← 5→ | 0.33 | −5 | ←−5→ | 0.07 | 0 |
| RV | 1.5 | −18 | 0.06 | ← 2→ | | −20 | ←−20→ | | 0 |

Boldface data: actual measured values (all other values calculated from them).

$P_{TP}$ = Transpulmonary pressure = Column B − Column D = Column F − Column D. This is the net inflation pressure of the lungs.

$P_{TC}$ = Transchestwall pressure = Column F − Column I = Column G. This is the net inflation pressure of the thoracic wall (rib cage, diaphragm, abdominal contents and anterior abdominal wall).

$C_T$ = Compliance of the total respiratory system = $\dfrac{\Delta\ \text{Column A}}{\Delta\ (\text{Col. B−I})} = \dfrac{\Delta\ \text{Volume}}{\Delta\ \text{Transtotal pressure}}$.

$C_L$ = Compliance of the lung = $\dfrac{\Delta\ \text{Column A}}{\Delta\ \text{Column D}} = \dfrac{\Delta\ \text{Volume}}{\Delta\ \text{Transpulmonary pressure}}$.

$C_{CW}$ = Compliance of the chest wall = $\dfrac{\Delta\ \text{Column A}}{\Delta\ \text{Column G}} = \dfrac{\Delta\ \text{Volume}}{\Delta\ \text{Transchestwall pressure}}$.

$\dfrac{1}{C_T} = \dfrac{1}{C_L} + \dfrac{1}{C_{CW}}$; Column B = Column D + Column G.

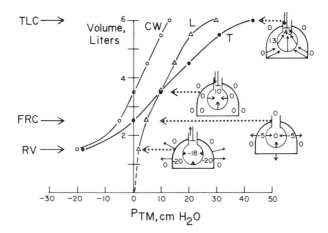

**FIG. 5.** Volume vs transmural pressure of the lungs (L), the chestwall (CW), and the total system (T) are plotted on the same axes. At TLC, at the equilibrium volume of the chestwall, at FRC, and at RV diagrams have been drawn to show the pressures in the alveoli and in the intrapleural space (PB stays zero). Also in the diagrams, *arrows* have been drawn to show the direction of and give an idea of the magnitude of the elastic pulls of the lungs and chestwall at the various volumes.

## THE LUNG CURVE

As one deflates the system from TLC to RV, the lungs (L) are fairly stiff initially (their compliance is fairly low initially), as demonstrated by the fairly low $\Delta V/\Delta P_{TP}$ during the first half-liter of deflation. From there on down to a little below FRC, their compliance is approximately constant at 0.2 liter/cm $H_2O$. Near RV, their compliance gets quite large, and the dotted line from RV down to the equilibrium volume of the lungs shows that the CL would get even higher if it were possible to deflate the system below RV *in vivo.*

## THE CHESTWALL CURVE

During the deflation from TLC to RV, the passive chestwall (CW) exhibits a quite constant compliance of 0.2 liter/cm $H_2O$ between TLC and FRC. Its compliance falls off (it gets stiffer) between FRC and RV. The passive chestwall passes through its equilibrium point at about FRC + 1 liter (3.5 liters). At that volume the passive chestwall is neither stretched nor compressed, and develops no transmural pressure across itself.

## THE TOTAL SYSTEM CURVE

The total system (T) has a relatively low compliance near TLC (like the lungs) and also between FRC and RV (like the chestwall), but a higher and constant compliance throughout the midrange (like both of its component parts). That constant compliance in the midrange is 0.1 liter/cm $H_2O$, or one-half of the compliance of either lungs or chestwall; in other words, the total system is twice as stiff as either of its components. This makes sense because inflating or deflating the total system compares to inflating or deflating one of its components alone, as inflating two concentric balloons compares to inflating only one. A greater pressure change must be exerted to cause a given volume change in the two concentric balloons than is needed to cause that volume change in the one balloon. (I have been known to use the "hot-air" power of one of my more verbal students to make this point!) It makes sense also because one must add compliances in series reciprocally to find the total compliance. Thus, $1/C_T = 1/C_L + 1/C_{CW} = 1/0.2 + 1/0.2 = 2/0.2$; $C_T = 0.1$ liter/cm $H_2O$. As is shown in Table 1, and can be seen in Fig. 5, $P_{TT}$ at any given volume must be algebraically equal to the sum of $P_{TP}$ and $P_{TC}$.

## INTERACTION BETWEEN LUNGS AND CHESTWALL

The diagrams to the right of Fig. 5 show the pressures ($P_A$, $P_{IP}$, and $P_B$) at each of four volumes during the deflation of the respiratory system. They also show the elastic recoil tendencies of the lungs and chestwall at each of those four volumes through the use of arrows emanating from lungs and chestwall.

At FRC, $P_{IP} = -5$ cm $H_2O$, while both $P_A$ and $P_B = 0$ cm $H_2O$. There is thus no difference in pressure across the whole system at this volume, which defines this as the equilibrium volume for the whole system, the volume to which the system returns when neither the respiratory muscles nor outside forces are pushing or pulling on the system. At this volume $P_{TP} = +5$ cm $H_2O$ and $P_{TC} = -5$ cm $H_2O$, equal and opposite; the arrows show that the lungs' elastic recoil is tending to collapse them just as strongly as the chestwall's elastic recoil is tending to expand it. In other words, the chestwall is pulling just as hard toward TLC as the lungs are pulling toward RV, and the system is in balance. The $P_{IP}$ of $-5$ cm $H_2O$ at FRC is thus generated by the tendency of the lungs and chestwall to pull away from one another.

The whole passive system can be held at a volume greater than FRC if either the $P_A$ is held greater than $P_B$ or the pressure outside the chest is held less than $P_B$. In the two such examples shown in Fig. 5, $P_A$ was held greater than $P_B$ by means of some sort of pump, here shown as a large syringe. When $P_A$ is raised to $+10$ cm $H_2O$ and held there, the volume of the whole system stays at 3.5 liters. At this volume the chestwall is at its equilibrium volume and thus needs no difference in pressure across it to keep it there ($P_{TC} = O$; $P_{IP} = P_B$), and the transpulmonary pressure equals the transtotal pressure of $+10$ cm $H_2O$ (the lung curve crosses the total curve). At this volume the lungs' elastic forces are pulling toward RV twice as strongly as they were at FRC; that pull is balanced by keeping the pressure inside the lungs $+10$ cm $H_2O$

greater than the pressure outside the lungs. When $P_A$ is raised to 43 cm $H_2O$ and held there, the volume of the whole system will be held at TLC. Here the lungs are stretched quite a lot and their elastic characteristics generate a very strong pull toward RV. That pull is balanced by a pressure difference across the lungs of +30 cm $H_2O$ ($P_A$ is +30 cm $H_2O$ greater than $P_{IP}$, and thus $P_{TP}$ = +30 cm $H_2O$). At this volume the chestwall also is much larger than its equilibrium volume, and its elastic characteristics generate a pull toward RV. That pull is balanced by $P_{TC}$ = 13 cm $H_2O$. At this volume, $P_{TT}$ = $P_{TP}$ + $P_{TC}$ = (+30) + (+13) = +43 cm $H_2O$.

The whole passive system can be held at a volume below FRC if $P_A$ is held below $P_B$. In the example shown in Fig. 5, the system was held at RV by holding $P_A$ at −18 cm $H_2O$. At this volume, the lungs are only slightly stretched, their tendency to deflate being balanced by $P_{TP}$ = +2 cm $H_2O$ [$P_{TP}$ = $P_A$ − $P_{IP}$ = (−18) − (−20) = +2 cm $H_2O$]. The chestwall is very much smaller than its equilibrium volume and causes its elastic characteristics to pull strongly toward TLC, that tendency being balanced by a large negative transchestwall pressure [$P_{TC}$ = $P_{IP}$ − $P_B$ = (−20) − (0) = −20 cm $H_2O$]. $P_{TT}$ again is equal to $P_{TP}$ + $P_{TC}$ = (+2) + (−20) = −18 cm $H_2O$.

I would again like to emphasize that all the compliance data so far discussed have been obtained under static conditions—no flow while measurements were being made.

## SPECIFIC COMPLIANCE

How does the compliance of the lungs of a mouse compare with the compliance of the lungs of an elephant? How do the compliances of newborn and adult human lungs compare? How does the compliance of one lobe of one human lung compare with the compliance of the two human lungs together?

These questions suggest a difficulty in comparing elastic characteristics of lungs or chestwalls of differing size. You already know that the $C_L$ of a normal, healthy person is about 0.2 liter/cm $H_2O$ in the midrange. The $C_L$ of one of the lobes of the right lung of a normal, healthy human may be about 0.03 liter/cm $H_2O$, whereas the $C_L$ of a normal newborn may be only 0.0045 liter/cm $H_2O$. This does not necessarily mean that the tissues of the lung of a normal newborn are stiffer than those of an adult, and it certainly doesn't mean that the adult right lung lobe has stiffer tissues than the lung as a whole. What it does mean is that the values of compliance must be normalized by relating them to the size of the lung (or part of the lung) in each case. One way in which this has been accomplished is by dividing $C_L$ by FRC, and this figure has been called "specific compliance." Using this procedure, the specific $C_L$ of the normal adult human is (0.2 liter/cm $H_2O$)/2.5 liters = 0.08/cm $H_2O$, whereas the specific $C_L$ of the normal newborn is (0.0045 liter/cm $H_2O$)/0.08 liter = 0.06/cm $H_2O$, a very similar figure. In fact, Schmidt-Nielsen has compared the compliances of the respiratory systems of a wide range of mammals and his figures enable one to calculate specific $C_L$ of about 0.08/cm $H_2O$ for the whole size spectrum of mammals from bat to whale.

## WHAT DETERMINES ELASTIC CHARACTERISTICS OF CHESTWALL AND LUNGS?

Chestwall compliance depends on the rigidity of the thoracic cage and on its shape. Thus, $C_{CW}$ may be decreased in arthritic spondylitis and extreme obesity, and in kyphoscoliosis and pectus excavatum. Chestwall compliance also depends on the diaphragm and abdominal structures, which represent one component of the chestwall. Thus, $C_{CW}$ may be decreased in abdominal disorders characterized by marked elevation of the diaphragm, or by skeletal muscle disorders associated with spasticity or rigidity of the thoracic or abdominal musculature. Lung compliance depends on the elastic characteristics of the lung tissue itself, and on the surface tension generated by the air–liquid interface at the alveolar surface. This information was set forth very clearly by Von Neergard in 1929, who concluded, "The total retraction of the lungs is divided into two components; the more important component is the action of surface tension, while true tissue elasticity is less important." Because he realized that two-thirds to three-quarters of the elastic recoil of adult lungs was caused by surface tension, Von Neergaard also understood that the sudden appearance of a subatmospheric pressure in the pleural space of the neonate was probably caused by the coincident generation of an air–liquid interface at the alveolar surface. These insights, published in the German literature, were largely ignored by pulmonary physiologists until the 1950's.

In 1957, Radford presented some experimental results obtained from studies similar to those of Von Neergaard almost 30 years before. It is only because Radford plotted his results in the more currently familiar form that his data are presented in Fig. 6 rather than those of Von Neergaard. The graph compares the volume versus $P_{TP}$ curves of a cat lung as stepwise inflation followed by stepwise deflation was performed with saline, on the one hand, and with air, on the other. Two important conclusions can be drawn immediately from the graph. Firstly, the saline inflation and deflation generates a far steeper slope than does the air inflation and deflation. When deprived of their air–liquid interface, the lungs are far less stiff, or far more compliant, than they are when it is present (remember, $C_L = (\Delta V)/(\Delta P_{TP})$). Said still another way, when the air–liquid interface was eliminated by the saline, most of the elastic recoil of the lungs was eliminated as well. Secondly, there is much more hysteresis between the air filling and emptying curves than there is between the saline filling and emptying curves. That is, the filling and emptying curves are almost coincident when the air–liquid interface is eliminated, but take widely different paths when it is present. It is worth pointing out that this extreme hysteresis is only seen

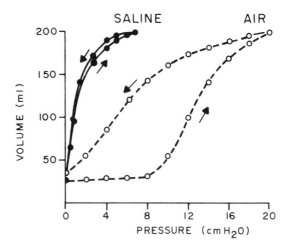

**FIG. 6.** Volume vs inflation pressure during lung inflation with air and with saline. Compliance is greater with saline. (Reproduced with permission from ref. 3, Clements, J. A.: Surface phenomena in relation to pulmonary function. *Physiologist,* 5:11, 1962.)

on the first inflation with air from a gas-free, or almost gas-free, state. Subsequent inflations and deflations lead to a less and less exaggerated difference between inflation and deflation, although some hysteresis exists even *in vivo.*

It may come as a surprise to the beginning student of pulmonary physiology that surface forces play so much of a part in determining the mechanical characteristics of the lungs. A brief consideration of the basic physics of surface forces, however, leads to other, rather surprising questions, such as, "How are we able to keep our alveoli open at all?" "How are alveoli of different sizes able to coexist simultaneously?" "What special problems does an infant experience during the traumatic transition between intra- and extrauterine life, between liquid breathing and air breathing?" Let us now consider surface tension and its role in the lung.

## SURFACE TENSION

Anyone who has ever tried to pull two wet microscope slides apart (not slide them apart) knows that surface tension can generate considerable forces. (The slides can be pulled apart easily while they are under water, however.) That surface tension can generate force can also be demonstrated by the Maxwell frame, shown in Fig. 7. A film of liquid is bounded by the U-shaped frame and its crossbar. The surface tension pulls the crossbar toward the end of the "U," and one must exert an equal and opposite force to prevent it from moving. That force, divided by the length of the bar in contact with the film, is the surface tension. If the force is 144 dynes, and the length is 1 cm, the surface

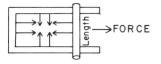

**FIG. 7.** The Maxwell frame to aid the conceptualization of the relationship among force (f), surface tension (T), and length (L). For a flat surface, T = f/L.

tension is 72 dynes/cm, the surface tension of an air–water interface. (There are two air–liquid interfaces here.)

When we consider surface tension in curved structures, a balance must be struck between tension and pressure. For example, a soap bubble can exist for some time, floating about without appreciable change in size. The surface tension, acting as an elastic film, squeezes the gas within the bubble, thus raising its pressure. The pressure difference thus generated (greater pressure inside than outside) exerts force directed outward, keeping the bubble from collapsing. The tension forces tending to collapse the bubble must be balanced by the pressure forces tending to make it expand, if the bubble size is to be kept constant. Figure 8 demonstrates this situation. Here, a plane and a hemisphere are being held together by the surface tension, which acts all along their common circumference, and are being pushed apart by a pressure inside the structure, which is higher than that outside. Balancing these two forces in a structure that is neither blowing apart nor collapsing, we may set them equal to one another. Thus, the tension force = $T \times$ (circumference) = $T \times (2\pi r)$, and the pressure force = $P \times$ (area of common circle) = $P \times (\pi r^2)$. Equating $\pi r^2 P = 2\pi r T$, dividing both sides by $\pi r$, and rearranging, we get $P = 2T/r$, which is LaPlace's law for a sphere. Actually, the P is really a difference in P, the transmural pressure, or $P_{in} - P_{out}$, so that $P_{TM} = 2T/r$.

## SURFACE TENSION AT ALVEOLAR SURFACE

Obviously, the alveoli are not simply a collection of soap bubbles. The stretching of the fibers of which the lung parenchyma is constructed provides some of the recoil of the lung. The "solid" lung tissue also lends some stability to the alveolar architecture by preventing groups of alveoli from collapsing, a phenomenon called "interdependence." Surface tension, however, provides much of the lung's elastic recoil and is of major importance in maintaining alveolar stability. Let us thus "neglect the too, too, solid flesh," as Clements did in his

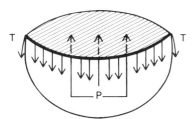

**FIG. 8.** The balance of forces generated by pressure and surface tension. The pressure, P, acting on the area of the plane tends to push the plane off the hemisphere. The tension, T, acting all along the circumference in common between the plane and hemisphere tends to hold the two together.

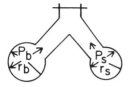

**FIG. 9.** For spheres, $P = 2T/r$. Thus, spheres having smaller radii (r) must develop greater transmural pressures ($P_s > P_b$) if their surface tensions (T) are equal. The small sphere must empty into the big one.

Bowditch lecture of 1961–1962, and consider the lungs to be an aggregate of air–liquid interfaces with spherical curvature.

We might begin by calculating what $P_{TM}$ would be needed to keep alveoli open at FRC in a normal human lung if the alveolar surface were like an air–saline interface, whose surface tension is about 72 dynes/cm. Assuming that there exists a population of alveoli whose radius is about $48 \times 10^{-4}$ cm at FRC, then $P_{TM} = 2T/r = 2(72$ dynes/cm$)/(48 \times 10^{-4}$ cm$) = 30 \times 10^3$ dynes/cm². If we remember that 1 cm $H_2O = 980$ dynes/cm², this $P_{TM}$ is about equal to 30 cm $H_2O$. Thus, if our assumptions were correct, the alveolar pressure would have to be 30 cm $H_2O$ greater than the intrapleural pressure at FRC, in a normal human lung. We already know from Fig. 5 and Table 1, however, that $P_{TP}$ at FRC in a normal human lung is only about 5 cm $H_2O$, one-sixth of what we just calculated. Since alveoli with radii of $48 \times 10^{-4}$ cm have been shown to exist in normal human lungs at FRC, it is our estimate of T which must be high by a factor of six. Thus, there must be a substance at the alveolar air–liquid interface that drastically lowers surface tension there.

This substance must do more than just keep T low. It must be capable of changing T as r changes. Consider an air–soap film interface, whose surface tension is low but constant regardless of whether the area of the film is increased or decreased. If we blow two bubbles of different sizes on a "Y" tube, as in Fig. 9, and then close the end of the tube, what happens? The smaller bubble will have a smaller radius ($r_s$) than the bigger one ($r_b$); thus, the same tension, T, will generate a larger $P_{TM}$ in the smaller bubble ($2T/r_s > 2T/r_b$). Since air moves from high to low pressure, the smaller bubble will empty into the larger one, faster and faster, as their radii become more and more disparate. In fact, given the same T in such a system, spheres of different sizes cannot coexist if connected to one another. Only if T were to change in the same direction as r, but faster than r changes, is stability possible. Only then could spheres with different radii develop the same $P_{TM}$ and thus coexist.

## WHAT IS THE SUBSTANCE LINING THE ALVEOLI AND HOW DOES IT WORK?

The substance that has been isolated in large quantities from the alveolar surface, and which seems to exhibit the same properties as the alveolar lining layer when spread on an aqueous surface, is dipalmitoyl phosphatidyl choline (DPPC). This material, whose structure is shown in Fig. 10, is quite unique.

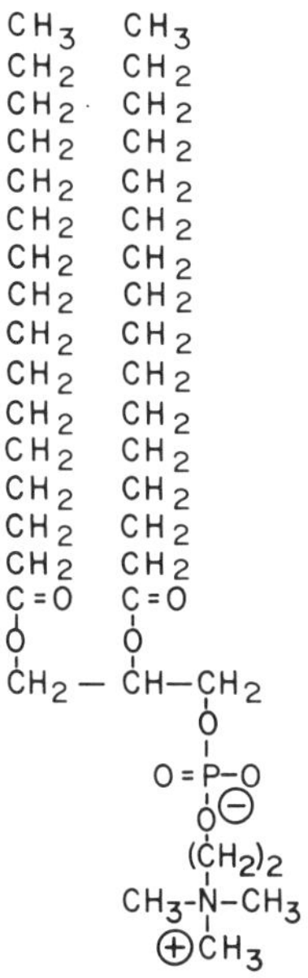

```
CH3   CH3
CH2   CH2
CH2·  CH2
CH2   CH2
CH2   CH2
CH2   CH2
CH2   CH2
CH2   CH2
CH2   CH2
CH2   CH2
CH2   CH2
CH2   CH2
CH2   CH2
CH2   CH2
CH2   CH2
C=O   C=O
 O     O
CH2 — CH—CH2
         O
      O=P–O
        O⊖
      (CH2)2
   CH3-N-CH3
     ⊕CH3
```

**FIG. 10.** The structure of DPPC. The two palmitate residues are oily, water insoluble, hydrophobic; the other end of the molecule is charged, water soluble, hydrophilic.

To the three carbons of a glycerol backbone are esterified two long-chain, straight (no double bonds) fatty acids and a phosphatidyl choline group. The nonpolar fatty acids, which are palmitate residues, are oily, bulky, and therefore hydrophobic ("water-hating"); in other words, that end of the molecule is essentially insoluble in water. The other, polar end of the molecule, being charged and relatively small, is hydrophilic ("water-loving") and dissolves easily in water. This molecule therefore orients perpendicularly to the surface of water, with its polar end dissolved and its nonpolar, bulky end sticking up. A monolayer of such molecules has considerable mechanical stability, due to the size and straightness of the nonpolar ends.

DPPC seems to work by generating a film pressure which opposes the surface tension of the air–saline interface. The three beakers in Fig. 11 schematize this concept. Beaker 1 shows simply an air–saline interface, which develops a surface tension of 72 dynes/cm. To the surface of beaker 2 have been added some molecules of DPPC, which are rather spread apart, and a barrier that is capable of sweeping across the surface of the saline, decreasing the area occupied by the DPPC, and thus compressing the film. The molecules of DPPC in beaker 2 are in a state similar to that of a few molecules of an ideal gas dispersed in a very large volume. The gas pressure would be essentially zero, as is the film pressure, and the surface tension would still be 72 dynes/cm. When the DPPC molecules are compressed together in beaker 3, however, their pressure (in two dimensions) increases just as does that of an ideal gas in three dimensions. If the compression is sufficient to raise the film pressure almost to 72 dynes/cm,

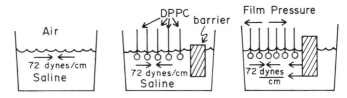

**FIG. 11.** Model of the mechanism by which DPPC reduces surface tension. The beaker on the left shows that an air–saline interface has a surface tension of 72 dynes/cm (or 72 mN/m). The beaker in the center holds molecules of DPPC and a surface barrier capable of crowding the DPPC together. Since the molecules of DPPC are still too far apart from one another to interact appreciably, the surface tension is still 72 dynes/cm. The beaker on the right shows that the DPPC, when crowded together, builds up a film pressure which counteracts some of the air–saline tension.

the surface tension of the interface will drop nearly to zero. Most films other than DPPC buckle, wrinkle, and break down before they can be compressed sufficiently to build up a film pressure of this magnitude, thus being unable to lower surface tension this much. DPPC, because of its mechanical stability, can lead to extremely low surface tensions both in beakers and in alveoli.

Just how low the surface tension *is* at the alveolar surface is a matter of some controversy. Based on indirect measurements from *in vitro* films and from volume–pressure data of excised lungs, Clements and others have concluded that it can approach zero as lung volume decreases (thus decreasing surface area and crowding DPPC molecules together). Other evidence has indicated that surface tension doesn't fall below about 18–20 dynes/cm, and some workers have suggested that surface active material is unnecessary for lung stability. Recently, however, Schürch et al. have measured alveolar surface tension directly by deflating excised lungs stepwise as droplets of fluid of various known surface tensions are deposited on the alveolar surface and observed. When the surface tension of the droplet is less than that of the alveolar surface, it spreads into a "lens" configuration; when the droplet surface tension is greater than that of the alveolar surface, it remains spherical. Some of their data are shown in Table 2. One can see that the surface tension is 9 dynes/cm even at a lung volume of 62% of TLC, and presumably gets even lower at smaller lung volumes.

TABLE 2. *Lung volume–alveolar surface tension relationship*

| No. of lungs | No. of observations | % TLC (mean ± SEM) | Surface tension (dynes/cm) | Test fluid |
|---|---|---|---|---|
| 6 | 25 | 62 ± 1.2 | 9 | FC 72 |
| 7 | 31 | 71 ± 1.0 | 13 | FC 75 |
| 5 | 21 | 78 ± 1.6 | 16 | FC 40 |
| 4 | 18 | 87 ± 1.3 | 20 | Silicone oil |

Data from Schürch et al., ref. 5.

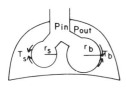

**FIG. 12.** How does DPPC stabilize alveoli in parallel? Again, $P_{TM} = 2T/r$, and alveoli with radii of different lengths cannot be kept inflated by the same P if their T are the same. If the $P_{TM}$ is sufficient to keep the big alveolus open, it can't keep the smaller one open if $T_b$ and $T_s$ are similar. So, the smaller alveolus begins shrinking. As it shrinks, its DPPC is crowded together, lowering its T drastically; and causing it to reach equilibrium with the existing $P_{TM}$.

The authors were unable to explore this latter possibility because they were unable to find a substance that had a surface tension lower than 9 dynes/cm and which would stay liquid at 37°C. It is now easy to see how different-sized alveoli could be stabilized by pulmonary surface active material (surfactant). Figure 12 shows two alveoli within the chest that are connected to one another by the airways. At any given moment, a certain pressure difference exists between the inside of the airways and alveoli, and the pleural space: $P_{TP} = P_A - P_{IP}$. This $P_{TP}$ is the same for both alveoli, but one has a small radius ($r_s$), and one has a big one ($r_b$). If we assume that the surface tension (T) starts out equal in the two alveoli, then this $P_{TP}$, if sufficient to keep the big alveolus open, cannot be large enough to keep the smaller one open (i.e., if $P_{TP} = 2T/r_b$, then $P_{TP}$ must be $< 2T/r_s$). Thus, the smaller alveolus begins to shrink. But as it does so, its surfactant molecules are crowded together raising the film pressure and decreasing the $T_s$. Since $T_s$ decreases faster than $r_s$, a state is automatically reached in which $P_{TP} = 2T_b/r_b = 2T_2/r_s$, and the two alveoli then require the same $P_{TP}$ to remain open.

## LONGER-TERM DYNAMIC CHARACTERISTICS OF SURFACTANT

If one compresses a film of DPPC sufficiently to produce very low T, and then keeps its area constant, T gradually rises with time toward about 25 dynes/cm. If one ventilates the lungs very shallowly, thus keeping the alveolar surface area almost constant, T also tends to rise toward some "equilibrium" value. It appears that the surfactant molecules, when compressed together tightly, tend to be squeezed out of the surface with time until their concentration is such that the tendency to enter the surface is equal to the tendency to be squeezed out of it. When Schürch et al. deflated excised lungs from TLC to approximately FRC and held them there, T rose above 9 dynes/cm after about 30 minutes. So, *constant—or nearly constant—surface area is not good for lungs.* Normal people, after a period of quiet, shallow breathing, find that a deep sigh is reflexly generated. This inflation to large volume (and large area) spreads out the surfactant molecules, allows addition of further surfactant molecules to the air–liquid interface through a mechanism not yet well understood, and results in a nice low T when the molecules of surfactant are again crowded together at volumes near FRC. Patients who have undergone abdominal or thoracic surgery may tend to avoid inspiring deeply because they find it painful.

They must be strongly urged to do so periodically, in order to avoid closing of lung units and resultant infection.

Workers in the field now seem to agree that the alveolar type II cells are the site of manufacture of surfactant, and they have measured its approximate rate of production. However, the mechanisms by which deep inspiration causes surfactant molecules to be added to the alveolar surface are poorly understood at best, and the mechanisms that remove and/or destroy surfactant have yet to be studied effectively.

During the intrauterine life of the fetus, of course, there is no air–liquid interface, and no necessity for surfactant. The mature fetus "breathes" amniotic fluid, maintaining a lung volume about at FRC. The transition to air breathing must be preceded by the development of the machinery capable of generating an appropriate alveolar lining layer. The maturation of this machinery normally seems to occur very late in pregnancy. DPPC first appears on the fetal alveolar surface at about 25 weeks of gestation, and reaches high concentrations at about 32–36 weeks (term is about 40 weeks). Occasionally, for any number of reasons including maternal diabetes mellitus; periods of fetal hypoperfusion in the immediate prenatal period; and most importantly, prematurity, infants are born with an immature alveolar lining layer. This condition, which has been termed, *Respiratory Distress Syndrome* of the newborn (RDS), affects some 30,000–50,000 newborns per year in the USA, and is characterized by T being high and not changing greatly with change in area. Figure 13 compares the area versus T curves of lung extracts from infants dying from non-RDS conditions with those from RDS infants. The T of the former group's extract varies from about 45 dynes/cm, when the area is maximum (100%), to less than 5 dynes/cm, when area is at a minimum (20%), and the curves exhibit considerable hysteresis.

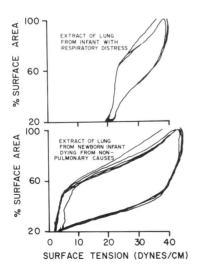

FIG. 13. Surface tension of lung extracts. **Bottom:** Extract from normal lung; minimal surface tension (after compresssion of film to 20% of original surface) = 2 dynes/cm. **Top:** Extract from lung of a newborn baby who died of RDS of the newborn; minimal surface tension = 20 dynes/cm. [Reproduced with permission from ref. 3, Clements, J. A.: Surface phenomena in relation to pulmonary function. *Physiologist,* 5:11, 1962 (data of W. H. Tooley).]

The T of the RDS group varies only between about 45 and 20 dynes/cm, and the curves exhibit much less hysteresis.

This abnormal alveolar lining layer causes grave problems for the newborn. Firstly, the high T means stiff lungs (low compliance). While a normal-term newborn has a lung compliance of about 4.5 ml/cm $H_2O$, the RDS newborn may have a $C_L$ of only 0.5 ml/cm $H_2O$. The infant must expend an inordinate amount of energy just to expand these lungs and, as soon as the respiratory muscles stop their inspiratory effort, the very stiff lungs tend to quickly deflate to very low volumes. Secondly, the small change in T with change in area means that different-sized alveoli are not stabilized as they normally would be. Thus, many—especially smaller—units become airless after each inspiration, the blood perfusing these units becoming a right-to-left (R-L) shunt. Thirdly, a pink, fibrinous thickening of the alveolar membranes may occur (leading to the alternate name, Hyaline Membrane Disease) which hinders gas diffusion between blood and gas. Because of these dysfunctions, the infant becomes hypoxic, hypercapnic, acidotic, and exhausted. Whether the infant lives or dies depends on the outcome of the race between worsening gas exchange on the one hand, and maturation of the surfactant manufacturing machinery on the other.

Two decades ago, that was all there was to the story. One simply waited out the race, giving $O_2$ and fluids. The outcome was clear in 72 hours, and the odds were about 50/50. Research has made the picture very much brighter today. The physician can, and does in some cases, sample amniotic fluid near term to determine if the surfactant machinery is mature. If it is not, or even without that test if the case history suggests high risk, the physician can delay delivery while accelerating the maturity of the machinery. Beta-adrenergic agonists and ethyl alcohol have been used to delay delivery, and glucocorticoids such as dexamethasone have been used to hasten maturity of the surfactant machinery. Even when an infant is born with RDS, his chances of survival at a major medical center are much improved. Treated with continuous positive pressure respiration (CPPR) to partially counteract the high elastic recoil and to keep many more units open, 80–90% of such infants survive with essentially no sequellae to carry into adult life.

## DYNAMICS—RESISTANCE TO FLOW

Thus far we have dealt with static situations—without motion. Now we must consider the additional pressure differences needed to overcome resistance to flow. Although there is some small pulmonary tissue resistance normally, by far the largest resistive impedance that must be overcome during breathing is that due to the resistance to airflow. Figure 14 demonstrates that inspiratory flow in a spontaneously breathing person is accomplished as the chestwall is enlarged, enlarging the lung and decompressing its gas. The alveolar gas pressure, $P_A$, thus drops below atmospheric pressure, $P_B$, causing the flow of gas down

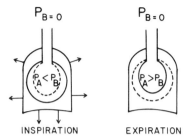

FIG. 14. Inspiration occurs by virtue of the alveolar gases being decompressed, thus lowering alveolar pressure (PA) below atmospheric pressure (PB). Expiration occurs when PA rises above PB.

$$P_B - P_A = \dot{V} \cdot R$$

its pressure gradient into the alveoli. Expiratory flow occurs as the respiratory muscles relax, allowing the lungs and chestwall to recoil toward FRC, thus compressing the alveolar gas and raising PA above PB. In both inspiration and expiration, a difference in pressure (here, a driving pressure) causes flow of gas through a resistance (here, the airway resistance). Airway resistance at rest in a normal person is about 1.5–2.5 cm $H_2O$/(liters/sec), depending on whether he is breathing through mouth or nose. Thus, since normal quiet breathing involves peak flows of about 0.5 liter/sec, the PA becomes about 1 cm $H_2O$ less than PB during inspiration, and about 1 cm $H_2O$ greater than PB during expiration (remember Ohm's law: $\Delta P = F \times R$, or $\Delta P = \dot{V} \times R$). Of course exercise, with its much higher flow rates, will involve much greater fluctuations of PA.

Let us now try to put together some of the compliance information with some of the airway resistance information. Suppose the following measurements were recorded from a person at rest, between breaths and therefore at FRC: PIP = −5 cm $H_2O$, CL = Ccw = 0.2 liter/cm $H_2O$, and airway resistance (RAW) = 2.0 cm $H_2O$/(liter/sec) during quiet breathing. Suppose this person then inspires all the way to TLC: What would be the values of PA and PIP just as he inspires past FRC + 1 liter at a flow rate of 1 liter/sec? First, knowing that PA must be lower than PB, we can calculate PB − PA = $\dot{V} \times$ RAW = (1 liter/sec) [2 cm $H_2O$/(liter/sec)] = 2 cm $H_2O$. Therefore, PA = −2 cm $H_2O$. We now need to find out what PTP must be at this volume. We know the initial PTP because we know the initial PIP; and we know that initially the person was between breaths, and that PA would therefore be equal to PB. Thus, initially, PTP = PA − PIP = 0 − (−5) = +5 cm $H_2O$. PTP will increase as the lung is made 1 liter larger. Knowing that CL = 0.2 liter/cm $H_2O$, and that CL = $\Delta V/\Delta$PTP, or $\Delta$PTP = $\Delta V/$CL, we can calculate $\Delta$PTP = 1 liter/(0.2 liter/cm $H_2O$) =+5 cm $H_2O$. The transpulmonary pressure was initially +5 cm $H_2O$ and has now increased by +5 cm $H_2O$ to become +10 cm $H_2O$. PTP = PA − PIP, and PIP = PA − PTP = −2 cm $H_2O$ − (+10 cm $H_2O$) =

−12 cm $H_2O$. The initial state of the system and its state as it passes through FRC + 1 liter are shown in Fig. 15.

Thus far we have assumed that airway resistance and lung compliance are independent of one another, and further, that airway resistance is constant and quantifiable through the use of Ohm's law. As is so often the case in physiology, neither of these simplifying assumptions is strictly true.

The second assumption is untrue because airflow in the tracheobronchial tree may become turbulent in some of the larger airways, rather than laminar (in straight lines parallel to the walls). The driving pressure required to cause flow through a given tube depends on the flow squared in turbulent flow, whereas it depends on the flow in laminar flow. Thus, the driving pressure, ΔP needed to cause a given air flow will really depend on flow and flow squared as in Rohrer's equation: $\Delta P = K_1(\dot{V}) + K_2(\dot{V}^2)$. Fortunately, the second component is rather small during quiet breathing, and the equation reduces to Ohm's law, $\Delta P = K_1 (\dot{V})$, where $K_1 = R$.

The first assumption is untrue because the elastic recoil of the lungs helps keep the intrathoracic airways open, as shown in Fig. 15. There is a transmural pressure difference of +5 cm $H_2O$ between PAW and PIP at FRC, tending to distend the intrathoracic airways. During inspiration the transmural pressure gets even greater, here shown to be 10–12 cm $H_2O$, and the opposite tends to happen during expiration. If the lungs were more compliant (less stiff, less elastic recoil), there would be a less subatmospheric PIP under all conditions, less transmural pressure to distend the airways, and a higher airway resistance, especially during expiration.

Using the expiratory muscles to raise PIP above atmospheric, in an attempt to speed up expiration, turns out to be an exercise in futility because the high PIP acts to collapse intrathoracic airways, and thus raises airway resistance. Under these conditions, flow proceeds only to the extent that the internal pressure exceeds the external pressure on the walls of the tube. Remember that the C-shaped rings of the trachea permit the dorsal soft tissue to bulge in and occlude the lumen. Fortunately, any increase in PIP is transmitted to increase PA; however, PA is raised above PIP only by virtue of the elastic recoil of the lungs,

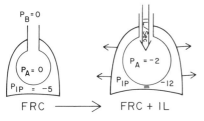

FIG. 15. The pressures in a normal person's respiratory system at FRC, and then again during inspiration toward TLC at a constant flow rate of 1 liter/sec. The picture on the *right* is a "snapshot" taken just as the person's lung volume passes FRC + 1 liter.

which also tends to compress the lung gas. Since the pressure increment produced by the elastic recoil of the lungs is a function of the lung volume, it will be large near TLC and much smaller near RV. Thus, in a forced expiration from full inspiration, there will come a point at which flow depends simply on lung volume and is independent of further increases in muscular effort (which raises alveolar pressure and collapsing pressure on the airways equally and therefore cancels out). For this reason also, expiratory flow is rapid at high lung volumes but gets progressively smaller as the lungs empty. Eventually, it stops completely from closure of all the airways and lack of elastic recoil to force air out through them. This is particularly true in older persons and in persons with some pulmonary diseases who have very compliant lungs, in whom RV is determined by closure of the airways and inability to force any more gas out of the lungs despite muscular effort.

This concept of expiratory flow limitation and its relationship to lung compliance is difficult for the beginning student to grasp but is very important. Therefore I believe it worthwhile to present it in more than one way. Figure 16 compares the pressures that might occur during a forced expiration from FRC + 3 liters in a normal person with those pressures in a person with severe emphysema and very compliant lungs. In both cases, the expiratory muscles have built up an intrapleural pressure of +20 cm $H_2O$. The normally stiff lungs on the left have added 15 cm $H_2O$ to produce an alveolar pressure of +35 cm $H_2O$ (PTP at this volume is +15 cm $H_2O$). The pressure difference, with PA being 35 cm $H_2O$ greater than PB, results in rapid expiratory flow of gas through the airway resistance with attendant drops in pressure along the path of the gas flow. Since the stiff lungs have added "lots" of pressure to that generated by

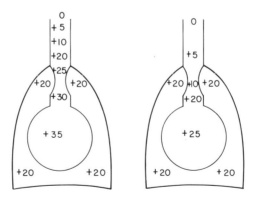

**FIG. 16.** Comparison of the pressures that might occur during a forced expiration in a normal person **(left)** with those pressures that might occur during forced expiration in an emphysematous person **(right)**. The intraairway pressures of the normal person are greater than his intrapleural pressures at this lung volume, and his airways therefore remain open. Because the flabby lungs of the emphysematous person add so little to his alveolar pressure, his intraairway pressure falls below his intrapleural pressure while the airways are still intrathoracic, leading to collapse.

the expiratory muscles, the airway pressure stays above the intrapleural pressure at all points in the intrathoracic airway, and no collapse occurs. Contrast this situation with that in the picture on the right of Fig. 16. The expiratory muscles have again built up a PIP of +20 cm $H_2O$, but these "flabby," too compliant lungs add only 5 cm $H_2O$ to this, which results in a PA of just +25 cm $H_2O$. Again, flow proceeds along the pressure difference, resulting in resistive pressure drops along the airway. In this case, however, the intraairway pressure falls below PIP well before the airway leaves the thorax, resulting in airway collapse. With airway collapse, the flow stops and the intraairway pressure rises to equal PA, which opens the airways. This sequence repeats itself over and over again, leading to a vibration called a "wheeze."

A useful test of pulmonary function is the measurement of the percentage of the vital capacity that a patient can expire in one second, or the peak expiratory flow that he can achieve. Either airway blockage (as from bronchiolar constriction) or low elastic recoil (as in severe emphysema) will slow the flow. At the bedside, one can simply ask the patient to try to blow out a match without pursing his lips or using his cheeks. The patient with severe emphysema and low elastic recoil of his lungs is unlikely to be able to blow it out. This inability makes it difficult for such patients to cough effectively. They thus have difficulty maintaining airway hygiene, and chronic infections may exacerbate their pulmonary disease.

## REFERENCES

1. Agostoni, E., and Mead, J. (1964): Statics of the respiratory system. In: *Handbook of Physiology, Sect. 3: Respiration,* edited by W. O. Fern and H. Rahn, Vol. 1, pp. 387–409. American Physiological Society, Washington, D.C.
2. Agostoni, E., and Mead, J. (1964): Dynamics of breathing. In: *Handbook of Physiology, Sect. 3: Respiration,* edited by W. O. Fern and H. Rahn, Vol. 1, pp. 411–427. American Physiological Society, Washington, D.C.
3. Clements, J. A. (1962): Surface phenomena in relation to pulmonary function. *Physiologist,* 5(1):11–28.
4. Goerke, J. (1974): Lung surfactant. *Biochem. Biophys. Acta,* 344:241–261.
5. Schürch, S., Goerke, J., and Clements, J. A. (1976): Direct determination of surface tension in the lung. *Proc. Natl. Acad. Sci. (USA),* 73(12):4698–4702.

## PROBLEMS

1. Questions A–C refer to the graph in Fig. 17 of the volume–pressure relationships of lungs during their deflation. You are given that the mean alveolar radius is $60 \times 10^{-4}$ cm at $V_3$ and $40 \times 10^{-4}$ cm at $V_1$.

   A. Which of the curves could have come from normal lungs whose surface tension (T) changes significantly with changes in surface area?

   B. Which of the curves could have come from the lungs of an infant with RDS of the newborn whose T changes little with changes in surface area?

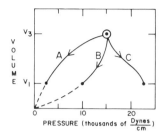

**FIG. 17.** Volume vs transpulmonary pressure during lung deflations.

C. Which of the curves could have come from lungs whose T doesn't change at all with changes in surface area?

2. Below is a list (a–e) of some possible properties of pulmonary surface active material. Which of the properties is responsible (or largely responsible) for the conditions stated in A–D?

### CONDITIONS

A. relatively low transpulmonary pressures needed to keep lungs inflated in normal people
B. relatively high lung compliance in normal people
C. coexistence of 300,000,000 alveoli of many different sizes
D. decrease in compliance during periods of quiet breathing

### PROPERTIES

a. changing surface tension with acutely changing surface area
b. change in rate of approach to equilibrium surface tension with change in temperature
c. tendency to approach an equilibrium surface tension when surface area is kept constant (or nearly constant)
d. ability to build up a high maximum film pressure
e. changing minimum surface tension with change in temperature

3. A man is paralyzed by poliomyelitis and his lungs are being ventilated by an iron lung. At FRC + 1 liter, in between inspiration and expiration while airflow is absent, $P_A = 0$, $P_{IP} = -10$, and the pressure outside the chest, in the respirator ($P_{RES}$) $= -15$ cm $H_2O$. The compliance of his lungs is 0.2 and that of his chest is 0.1 liter/cm $H_2O$.

A. At this volume (FRC + 1 liter), $P_{TC}$ is about
    a. $-5$ cm $H_2O$
    b. $0$ cm $H_2O$

   c. +5 cm $H_2O$
   d. +10 cm $H_2O$
   e. +15 cm $H_2O$

B. When he gets down to FRC and flow stops, PIP will be
   a. −15 cm $H_2O$
   b. −10 cm $H_2O$
   c. −5 cm $H_2O$
   d. 0 mm Hg
   e. +5 cm $H_2O$

C. When he gets down to FRC and flow stops, the transtotal pressure, PA
   − PRES, will be
   a. −10 cm $H_2O$
   b. −5 cm $H_2O$
   c. 0 cm $H_2O$
   d. +5 cm $H_2O$
   e. +15 cm $H_2O$

4. There is considerable difference between the minimum time it takes even a normal person to change his lung volume from RV to TLC and the minimum time it takes him to go from TLC to RV. The most probable explanation for this difference is that

   a. the chestwall tends to expand when the respiratory system is at RV
   b. the chestwall gets quite stiff near RV
   c. inspiratory muscles are capable of stronger efforts than expiratory muscles
   d. airways tend to collapse near RV during strong inspiratory efforts
   e. airways tend to collapse near RV during strong expiratory efforts

5. A completely paralyzed large person is lying with his body completely enclosed in a Drinker respirator ("iron lung"), while just his head and neck (including the opening of his tracheostomy tube) are sticking out into the room air. The tracheostomy tube has been inserted into the trachea below the larynx, and his airway is always unobstructed. Measurements of his respiratory mechanics produced the following values:

Transpulmonary pressure (PTP) at FRC with the respirator pressure at
atmospheric pressure         = 6 cm $H_2O$
Lung compliance (CL)        = 0.25 liters/cm $H_2O$
Chestwall compliance (CCW) = 0.20 liters/cm $H_2O$

   A. What respirator pressure would be needed to hold his lungs inflated to FRC + 0.5 liters?
   B. What would be his intrapleural pressure (PIP) under the conditions of A?

## ANSWERS

1. Merely calculate surface tension at the common point at $V_3$ (circled) and again at each final point at $V_1$, and you will find that it's as simple as ABC, i.e., curve A is consistent with the conditions stated in question **A,** curve B with those in question **B,** and curve C with those in question **C** ($P = 2T/r$).

2. **A:** Transpulmonary pressure will be low if surface tension is low. Surface tension will be low if film pressure is high. The pulmonary surface active material is one of the few substances capable of building up a film pressure sufficient to lower alveolar surface tension to 10 dynes/cm or less. Thus answer is (d).

   **B:** Same answer as in **A** for the same reasons.

   **C:** If surface tension were to remain constant, then small alveoli would close and empty into large ones (soap bubble demonstration) due to small radius yielding greater transmural pressure than large radius. Thus, the $3 \times 10^8$ alveoli coexist because surface tension changes in the same direction as radius but changes even faster than radius does. Thus, answer is (a).

   **D:** Answer is (c).

3. **A:** $P_{TC} = P_{IP} - P_{RES} = (-10) - (-15) = +5$ cm $H_2O$.

   **B and C:** The answers to these and other problems in physiology must be understood both intuitively and quantitatively. Intuitively, one should realize that the respiratory system is at equilibrium at FRC. Thus, if the airways are open and if the respiratory muscles are relaxed (they always are, in a paralyzed patient), the flow, $P_A$, and $P_{RES}$ must all be zero. Hence, the transtotal pressure, which is defined as $P_A - P_{RES}$ must be zero also.
   **B:** On a quantitative level, one should begin by drawing pictures of the situation at FRC + 1 liter, and the situation at FRC, and then proceed to fill in the blanks, working from pressures you know, across one barrier at a time, and calculating the next pressure from the compliance equation. The situation at FRC + 1 liter is shown in Fig. 18A, and Fig. 18B shows the situation at FRC when flow is zero. We need to calculate $P_{IP}$ and $P_{RES}$ in Fig. 18B. To calculate $P_{IP}$: $\Delta P_{TP} = \Delta V/C_L = -1$ liter/(0.2 liter/cm $H_2O$). Thus, $\Delta P_{TP} = -5$ cm $H_2O$. The original $P_{TP} = 0 - (-10) = +10$ cm $H_2O$. It has changed by $-5$ cm $H_2O$ and is thus now $+5$ cm $H_2O$. Since $P_A = 0$, the new $P_{IP}$ must be $-5$ cm $H_2O$. Thus, the answer is (c).
   **C:** This problem can be solved by continuing to work across the next barrier, using the compliance of the chestwall, or by considering the two barriers as one and using the compliance of the combined lung and chestwall. The latter approach is shown here. Adding the $C_L$ and $C_{CW}$ reciprocally gives $C_T = 1/15$ liter/cm $H_2O$. Then, the $\Delta P_{TT} = \Delta V/C_T = -1$ liter/(1/15

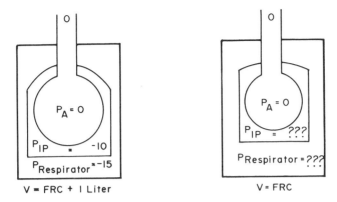

**FIG. 18.** Pressures within the respiratory system of a paralyzed patient in an iron lung at lung volumes of FRC + 1 liter and FRC. There is no gas flow taking place during the measurements in either case.

liter/cm $H_2O$) = −15 cm $H_2O$. $P_{TT}$ at FRC + 1 liter was +15 cm $H_2O$ and has changed by −15 cm $H_2O$. It is thus zero, as our intuition has suggested, and the answer is (c).

4. Answer is (e). Alternatives (a) and (b) are true but irrelevant, (c) and (d) are incorrect, which leaves (e) as the correct answer. Airways *do* tend to collapse near RV during strong expiratory efforts because, near RV, there is very little lung recoil tending to raise $P_A$. Thus, $P_A$ is only a little above $P_{IP}$; flow through the airways causes the usual drops in pressure due to resistance, and pressure within the thoracic airways drops below $P_{IP}$, causing their collapse.

5. **A:** The easiest way to get the answer to this problem is to calculate the change in $P_{TT}$ as a result of the $\Delta V$ of 0.5 liters, having determined $C_T$ by adding the individual compliances reciprocally. Thus: $1/C_L + 1/C_C = 1/C_T$, $1/C_T = 1/0.25 + 1/0.2 = 4 + 5 = 9$. If $1/C_T = 9$, $C_T = (1/9)$ liters/ cm $H_2O$. $\Delta P_{TT} = \Delta V/C_T = 0.5$ liters/(0.11 . . . liter/cm $H_2O$) = 4.5 cm $H_2O$. Since the person is paralyzed with an unobstructed airway, his $P_{TT}$ must have been 0 at FRC, and must now be +4.5 cm $H_2O$. As the respirator holds his lungs and chestwall at this new volume, $P_A$ must be 0, and $P_{RES}$ must thus be −4.5 cm $H_2O$.

**B:** Having calculated $P_{RES}$ for problem 5A, one can determine $P_{IP}$ at FRC + 0.5 liters by using the chestwall, or one can solve this problem independently from the previous one by using the lung. To use the lung, note that $P_{TP}$ at FRC was +6 cm $H_2O$, then calculate $\Delta P_{TP}$ as a result of the $\Delta V$ of 0.5 liters: $\Delta P_{TP} = 0.5$ liters/(0.25 liters/cm $H_2O$) = 2 cm $H_2O$. Thus, $P_{TP}$

must now be +8 cm $H_2O$, and since the PA must be 0 (as explained above), PIP must be −8 cm $H_2O$. To use the chestwall, first note that PTC was −6 cm $H_2O$ at FRC, then calculate ΔPTC as a result of the ΔV of 0.5 liters: ΔPTC = 0.5 liters/(0.2 liters/cm $H_2O$) = 2.5 cm $H_2O$. Thus, PTC must now be −6 + 2.5 = −3.5 cm $H_2O$. We can now calculate PIP using PTC and PRES: PTC = PIP − PRES, PIP = PTC + PRES = −3.5 +(−4.5) = −8 cm $H_2O$.

# 3

# *Ventilation and Alveolar Gas Pressures*

One of the tasks of the respiratory system is to adjust the flow of gas moving between the environment and the alveoli according to demands related to metabolism and environmental gas composition. This flow of environmental gas, having an oxygen partial pressure ($P_{O_2}$) greater than that in alveolar gas, and a $CO_2$ partial pressure ($P_{CO_2}$) less than that in alveolar gas, will tend to replace the $O_2$ that is constantly being removed from the alveolar gas by the blood and to carry away the $CO_2$ that is constantly being put into the alveolar gas. Clearly, for a given metabolic rate, a higher gas flow into the alveoli raises $P_{O_2}$ and lowers $P_{CO_2}$. In the steady state, by definition, neither the flow of gas nor the mean alveolar partial pressures of $O_2$ or $CO_2$ ($P_{A_{O_2}}$, $P_{A_{CO_2}}$) change appreciably with time. In fact, however, since breathing is intermittent, $P_{A_{CO_2}}$ and $P_{A_{O_2}}$ tend to vary above and below the mean values by a few millimeters of mercury, as seen in Fig. 1. Here the mean values of $P_{A_{CO_2}}$ and $P_{A_{O_2}}$ are about 39 and 100 mm Hg, respectively. Inspiration of $O_2$-rich and essentially $CO_2$-free gas raises $P_{A_{O_2}}$ and reduces $P_{A_{CO_2}}$ somewhat. Between the end of that inspiration and the next inspiration, the partial pressure of $O_2$ falls below and that of $CO_2$ rises above, the mean values, again just by a mm Hg or so, as exchange between gas and blood continues. The breath-to-breath changes in $P_{A_{CO_2}}$ and $P_{A_{O_2}}$ are so small because the volume of gas moved into the alveoli with each inspiration is small compared with the volume of gas already present. In a normal resting individual inspiration moves only about 0.35 liter of environmental gas into the alveoli with each breath, and the FRC is about 2.5 liters. We find it convenient to ignore these small variations for most purposes, and consider only the mean $P_{A_{CO_2}}$ and the mean $P_{A_{O_2}}$.

This chapter discusses the following concepts: (a) The definitions of and difference between total minute ventilation ($\dot{V}_I$ or $\dot{V}_E$) and alveolar ventilation ($\dot{V}_A$), involving definition of respiratory dead space ($V_D$) and its measurement; (b) the dependence of $P_{A_{CO_2}}$ on metabolic production of $CO_2$ ($\dot{V}_{CO_2}$) and alveolar ventilation ($\dot{V}_A$); (c) the dependence of $P_{A_{O_2}}$ on $P_{A_{CO_2}}$, $P_B$, fraction of $O_2$ in ⋅

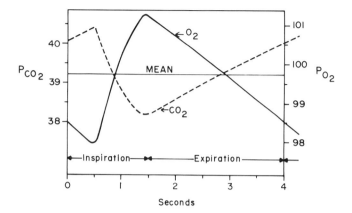

**FIG. 1.** Changes in alveolar $O_2$ and $CO_2$ during a normal respiratory cycle. The curves cross the line which identifies the mean alveolar values once during inspiration and once during expiration. [Reproduced with permission from Rahn, H. and Farhi, L.: Ventilation, perfusion, and gas exchange—the $\dot{V}A/\dot{Q}$ concept. In: *Handbook of Physiology, Sect. 3: Respiration,* edited by W. O. Fenn and H. Rahn, Vol. 1, p. 735. American Physiological Society, Washington, D.C., 1964.

inspired gas ($FI_{O_2}$), and respiratory exchange ratio (R); and (d) some of the practical uses of these relationships.

## TIDAL VOLUME ($V_T$)

Each respiratory cycle moves a volume of gas, the tidal volume ($V_T$), from the environment past the nose or mouth and into the respiratory system. Regardless of the temperature and water vapor content of the gas of the environment, the warm, moist passages of the respiratory system warm this inspired gas to body temperature ($\approx 37°C$) and saturate it with water vapor at this temperature $PH_2O = 47$ mm Hg). This process, essentially complete by the time the inspired gas has reached the trachea, usually results in an increase in volume since the environmental temperature and water vapor pressure are usually lower than the values of those variables in the respiratory trace. Since we are usually interested in the volume of gas actually moved by the respiratory system, $V_T$ is usually expressed in liters/breath, at Body Temperature, Pressure, and Saturated with water vapor (BTPS). The actual $V_T$, BTPS, can be measured with a body plethysmograph, but if $V_T$ is measured by some other means, the ideal gas laws can be used to convert the volume to BTPS conditions. Assume, for instance, that $V_T$ is 456.3 ml/breath, as averaged during several minutes of breathing to and from a spirometer whose temperature is 21°C and whose $PH_2O = 19$ mm Hg (saturated at 21°C). Assuming we are at sea level where the barometric pressure (PB) is 760 mm Hg, we can convert $V_T$ to $V_T$, BTPS, as follows:

$$\frac{P_1 V_1}{T_1} = \frac{P_2 V_2}{T_2}$$

$$V_2 = \frac{P_1 V_1 T_2}{T_1 P_2} = \frac{(741 \text{ mm Hg}) (456.3 \text{ ml/breath})(310°\text{K})}{(294°\text{K}) (713 \text{ mm Hg})} = 500 \text{ ml/breath}$$

## $\dot{V}$I and $\dot{V}$E. $\dot{V}$O₂, $\dot{V}$CO₂, and R.Q.

So, the respiratory system was moving 500 ml through the trachea with each breath. If the respiratory frequency (f) was 12 breaths/min, then the inspired minute ventilation ($\dot{V}$I) was 6,000 ml/min, BTPS. The expired minute ventilation ($\dot{V}$E) would ordinarily be slightly less than this because the respiratory quotient (R.Q.) is ordinarily somewhat less than 1. That is, the $CO_2$ production ($\dot{V}CO_2$) is normally slightly less than the oxygen consumption ($\dot{V}O_2$), those values in a basal person of normal size being, respectively, about 200 ml/min and 250 ml/min. [These values are ordinarily expressed as volumes/min, Standard Temperature and Pressure, Dry ($\dot{V}$, STPD), since only then are the volumes directly related to the number of moles of gas consumed or produced.] Under these conditions, $\dot{V}$E will be about 60.5 ml/min less than $\dot{V}$I, since the alveolar gas is losing more molecules of $O_2$ to the blood than it is gaining $CO_2$ molecules from the blood. (If your number differs from 60.5 ml, you probably forgot that $\dot{V}CO_2$ and $\dot{V}O_2$ are expressed under STPD conditions, whereas $\dot{V}$I and $\dot{V}$E are expressed under BTPS conditions.)

## VD and $\dot{V}$A

In this normal individual, the respiratory passages between external environment and alveoli have an internal volume of about 150 ml [the anatomic dead space (VD) ≅ 150 ml]. At the end of an expiration, these passages will have about 150 ml of alveolar gas left in them. During the next inspiration, this 150 ml of gas must be moved into the alveoli before any fresh environmental gas can arrive. Thus, although 500 ml of environmental gas may have moved past the nose or mouth, and 500 ml of gas will have moved into the alveoli, perhaps only 350 ml of *environmental* gas will have moved into the alveoli, and only in the alveoli is significant gas exchange possible. The volume of environmental gas that reaches the alveoli with each breath (VA) can then be calculated as VA = VT − VD; and the flow of environmental gas into the alveoli each minute ($\dot{V}$A) can be calculated as $\dot{V}$A = VA(f) = the alveolar ventilation. So, in this case, $\dot{V}$A = 350 ml/breath (12 breaths/min) = 4,200 ml/min, BTPS. I would emphasize here that only $\dot{V}$A, not the larger $\dot{V}$E or $\dot{V}$I, is effective in maintaining gas exchange in the lungs.

VD can be measured either by a "single-breath method" or by utilizing the Bohr equation. A determination of VD by the "single-breath method" is shown in Fig. 2. Here, the percentage of $N_2$ is measured continuously at the subject's mouth and is plotted on the ordinate, and the volume inspired and expired is plotted on the abscissa, as the subject takes a deep breath of pure $O_2$ and then exhales steadily. Prior to the breath of $O_2$, both the alveolar gas and inspired gas have 79% $N_2$. While $O_2$ is being inspired, the meter shows 0% $N_2$, and at the end of that inspiration, pure $O_2$ is left in the dead space. Thus, the percentage of $N_2$ in the exhaled gas is initially zero (VD expired first), and rises to a plateau as pure alveolar gas is finally exhaled. The percentage of $N_2$ doesn't rise as a square wave because there is mixing along the front between dead space gas and alveolar gas. If one then "squares off" the transition with a vertical line (as though there were no mixing) such that areas $A$ and $B$ are equal, and measures the volume exhaled until the vertical line, one has a measure of the anatomic dead space.

In respiratory disease, but not in health, there may be some alveoli that are not perfused at all, but which are ventilated nonetheless. This ventilation to nonperfused alveoli constitutes "wasted ventilation." This "wasted ventilation" together with the anatomic dead space constitute the "physiological dead space," or total dead space, and this volume can be measured using the Bohr equation. The procedure involves collecting the expired gas for a number of breaths,

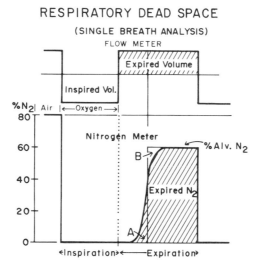

RESPIRATORY DEAD SPACE
(SINGLE BREATH ANALYSIS)

**FIG. 2.** Method of measuring anatomic dead space. *Ordinate:* Percentage of $N_2$ in inspired and expired gas. *Abscissa:* Volume of gas inspired (to *dotted line*) and expired (beyond *dotted line*). The subject takes a deep breath of pure $O_2$ and then exhales steadily. The percentage of $N_2$ in the expired gas is initially zero because of the inhalation of $O_2$. It rises sharply to a plateau when alveolar gas begins to be expired. A vertical line is drawn in such a way that $A$ and $B$ are equal. The distance along the abscissa between this line and the dotted line marking the start of expiration indicates the volume of gas that occupies the anatomic dead space. [Reproduced with permission from Comroe, J. H., Jr., et al.: *The Lung: Clinical Physiology and Pulmonary Function Tests,* 2nd Ed. Year Book Medical Publishers, Chicago, 1962.]

measuring the mixed expired $P_{CO_2}$ ($P_{ECO_2}$), and $V_T$, getting a good measure of $P_{ACO_2}$ in the perfused alveoli by measuring $P_{ACO_2}$, and then simply applying the principle of conservation of matter. Remember that the symbol F, as in $F_{ACO_2}$, refers to the fraction of *dry* gas molecules which are, in this case, $CO_2$ molecules; therefore $[P_{ACO_2}/(P_B - P_{H_2O})] = F_{ACO_2}$. So, since the $CO_2$ molecules which we have collected in the bag containing the expired gas all came from alveoli, we can calculate the physiological dead space as follows:

$$F_{ACO_2}(V_A) = F_{ECO_2}(V_T)$$

$$\frac{P_{ACO_2}(V_A)}{P_B - P_{H_2O}} = \frac{P_{ECO_2}(V_T)}{P_B - P_{H_2O}}$$

Multiplying through by $P_B - P_{H_2O}$ gives

$$P_{ACO_2}(V_A) = P_{ECO_2}(V_T)$$

or

$$V_A = \frac{P_{ECO_2}(V_T)}{P_{ACO_2}}$$

In our healthy person, $V_T$ might be 0.5 liter, and $P_{ECO_2}$ and $P_{ACO_2}$ might be, respectively, 28 and 40 mm Hg, so the volume involved in "good" alveolar exchange per breath would be 0.35 liter. Thus, as is usual in health, this person's "physiological" and anatomical dead spaces are both equal to 150 ml.

## FACTORS DETERMINING $P_{ACO_2}$

Now, having defined and learned how to measure $V_D$, let's just ignore it for a few moments and consider the lung to be a flow-through system as pictured in Fig. 3. The alveolar ventilation ($\dot{V}_A$) washes through these lungs at a constant

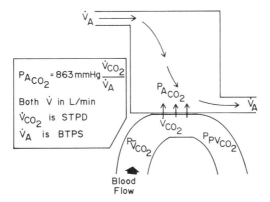

**FIG. 3.** A simple model of $CO_2$ exchange in the lungs.

rate. Remember that environmental gas usually contains essentially no $CO_2$. The question is, "upon what does $P_{A_{CO_2}}$ depend?" Clearly, higher $\dot{V}_{CO_2}$ (more molecules of $CO_2$ being put into the flowing stream of gas per minute) will result in a higher $P_{A_{CO_2}}$ by the time the gas leaves the lungs. The flowing stream of fresh gas (no $CO_2$) can be thought of as diluting the $CO_2$ in the alveolar gas. In this light, it is clear that lower $\dot{V}_A$, for any given $\dot{V}_{CO_2}$, will also raise $P_{A_{CO_2}}$. So qualitatively, $P_{A_{CO_2}}$ depends directly on $\dot{V}_{CO_2}$ and inversely on $\dot{V}_A$, in the steady state.

Let us now develop the quantitative relationship that can predict $P_{A_{CO_2}}$ in a steady state, again by using the principle of conservation of matter. First, $CO_2$ production is equal, in the steady state, to $CO_2$ elimination by the lungs, which is equal to the fraction of $CO_2$ in the alveolar gas times the alveolar ventilation, or, symbolically:

$$\dot{V}_{CO_2}, \text{STPD} = F_{A_{CO_2}}(\dot{V}_A, \text{STPD})$$

The only manipulations we need to make are to (a) the conversion of $F_{A_{CO_2}}$ to $P_{A_{CO_2}}$, and (b) the conversion of $\dot{V}_A$, STPD, to $\dot{V}_A$, BTPS, to deal with the volumes actually moved through the alveoli. To make the first manipulation, we simply multiply both sides of the equation by $P_B - P_{H_2O}$; and to make the second (using the ideal gas laws), we simply multiply both sides by

$$\frac{760 \text{ mm Hg}}{P_B - P_{H_2O}} \cdot \frac{310°K}{273°K}$$

to get the following:

$$(P_B - P_{H_2O}) \cdot \frac{760 \text{ mm Hg}}{(P_B - P_{H_2O})} \cdot \frac{310°K}{273°K} \cdot (\dot{V}_{CO_2}, \text{STPD}) = P_{A_{CO_2}}(\dot{V}_A, \text{BTPS})$$

Cancelling out $P_B - P_{H_2O}$, reducing the constant terms to one number, and rearranging, we get the final, useful form of the relationship:

$$P_{A_{CO_2}} = (863 \text{ mm Hg}) \frac{\dot{V}_{CO_2}, \text{STPD}}{\dot{V}_A, \text{BTPS}}$$

when both $\dot{V}_{CO_2}$ and $\dot{V}_A$ are in liters/time or milliliters/time. Knowing any two of the variables, one can calculate the third quantitatively in the steady state. From an initial steady state, the equation also tells which way $P_{A_{CO_2}}$ will change during the transient state, which is induced by changing one of the other two variables. Examples of steady state calculations are shown in Table 1, beginning with a resting, sea-level, control subject. Clinically, this relationship is extremely important, serving to give the physician a quick idea of the adequacy of a patient's alveolar ventilation. During anesthesia, for instance, the anesthesiologist may monitor airway $P_{CO_2}$ continuously with an infrared $CO_2$ analyzer, and thereby get a breath-by-breath measurement of $P_{CO_2}$ at the end of each expiration (when alveolar gas is being exhaled). If the $P_{A_{CO_2}}$ thus

TABLE 1. *Effect of changes in $\dot{V}_A$ and $\dot{V}_{CO_2}$ on steady-state $P_{A_{CO_2}}$*

| | $\dot{V}_{CO_2}$ (ml/min) | f (br/min) | $V_T$ (ml) | $V_D$ (ml/br) | $\dot{V}_E$ (ml/min) | $\dot{V}_A$ (ml/min) | $P_{A_{CO_2}}$ (mm Hg) |
|---|---|---|---|---|---|---|---|
| Control | 195 | 12 | 500 | 150 | 6,000 | 4,200 | 40 |
| Double f | 195 | 24 | 500 | 150 | 12,000 | 8,400 | 20 |
| Double $V_T$ | 195 | 12 | 1,000 | 150 | 12,000 | 10,200 | 16.5 |
| Both $\dot{V}_A$ and $\dot{V}_{CO_2} \times 10$ | 1,950 | | | | | 42,000 | 40 |

measured is 80 mm Hg, the anesthesiologist knows that the ratio of $\dot{V}_{CO_2}/\dot{V}_A$ is twice what it is in a normal resting man (let's assume that this patient had a normal $P_{A_{CO_2}}$ of about 40 mm Hg before being anesthetized). He knows that $\dot{V}_{CO_2}$ hasn't doubled. $\dot{V}_{CO_2}$ can be raised greatly by exercise, and by lesser amounts during fever or when hyperthyroidism is present. None of these factors should have raised $\dot{V}_{CO_2}$ in this case; in fact, anesthesia may even lower it. Thus, the anesthesiologist knows that $\dot{V}_A$ must be only about half what it should be, since $\dot{V}_{CO_2}$ is about normal, while $P_{A_{CO_2}}$ is doubled. In equation form: $P_{A_{CO_2}} (\dot{V}_A) = 863$ mm Hg $(\dot{V}_{CO_2})$. If, as in the case just discussed, there is no reason to suppose that $\dot{V}_{CO_2}$ has changed between one steady state and another, then $P_{A_{CO_2}} (\dot{V}_A) = 863$ mm Hg(K), or $P_{A_{CO_2}} (\dot{V}_A) = K'$, or $(P_{A_{CO_2}})_1$ $(\dot{V}_A)_1 = K' = (P_{A_{CO_2}})_2 (\dot{V}_A)_2$. If $(P_{A_{CO_2}})_2$ is twice what it was before, it must be because $(\dot{V}_A)_2$ is half what it was before.

We can generalize with the following statement: As $\dot{V}_A \rightarrow \infty$, $P_{A_{CO_2}}$ moves toward $P_{I_{CO_2}}$ (or, $\rightarrow 0$); as $\dot{V}_A \rightarrow 0$, $P_{A_{CO_2}}$ moves away from $P_{I_{CO_2}}$ (or, $\rightarrow \infty$). This hyperbolic relationship (XY = K) between $\dot{V}_A$ and $P_{A_{CO_2}}$ is plotted, for each of three constant $\dot{V}_{CO_2}$, in Fig. 4. The patient whose $\dot{V}_{CO_2}$ is essentially normal and unchanging from moment to moment moves along the bottom curve ($\dot{V}_{CO_2} = 0.2$ liter/min), his $P_{A_{CO_2}}$ related inversely to his $\dot{V}_A$. If the patient begins steady-state exercise, which raises his $\dot{V}_{CO_2}$ by a factor of five, he moves to the upper curve ($\dot{V}_{CO_2} = 1.0$ liter/min). If, as seems true for most people, his respiratory regulation is designed to keep $P_{A_{CO_2}}$ about the same in steady-state exercise as it is at rest, his new $\dot{V}_A$ is quite predictable given knowledge of his resting $\dot{V}_A$ or $P_{A_{CO_2}}$. Thus, in order to maintain a $P_{A_{CO_2}}$ of 43.15, his $\dot{V}_A$ must now be 20 liters/min.

## HYPERVENTILATION AND HYPOVENTILATION—DEFINITIONS

In fact, a common definition of hyperventilation and hypoventilation involves this relationship. A person is said to be "hyperventilating" if his ratio of $\dot{V}_{CO_2}/\dot{V}_A$ is lower than the norm for his sex, altitude of residence, etc., and to be "hypoventilating" if that ratio is higher than the norm. The ratio is about 1/21.6 for normal, resting, sea-level *men,* leading to the often quoted "normal" $P_{A_{CO_2}}$ of 40 mm Hg. Quoting this value as normal brands respiratory physiolo-

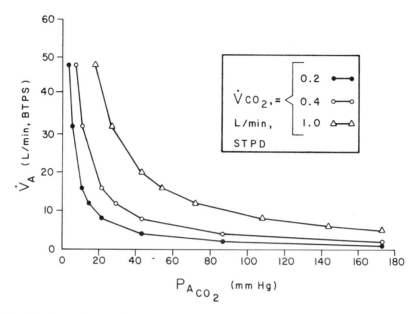

**FIG. 4.** Alveolar ventilation ($\dot{V}A$) vs alveolar $PCO_2$ ($PA_{CO_2}$) at each of three levels of $CO_2$ production ($\dot{V}CO_2$).

gists as not only "male chauvinist pigs," but "sea-level chauvinist pigs" as well! Women, probably due to their much higher levels of progesterone, run lower $PA_{CO_2}$ than men (about 36–37 mm Hg), and pregnant women (with even higher levels of progesterone) may run $PA_{CO_2}$ as low as 28–30 mm Hg. Either sex hyperventilates when made hypoxic, as at high altitude, and therefore may have considerably lower $PA_{CO_2}$ than would be expected at sea level. The subject of chemical regulation of ventilation will be dealt with in some detail in the last chapter of the respiration section of this book.

### FACTORS DETERMINING $PA_{O2}$

Qualitatively, the situation for $O_2$ is similar to that for $CO_2$ in that the blood continuously removes $O_2$ from the alveolar gas while alveolar ventilation periodically replaces it. Thus, as $\dot{V}A \twoheadrightarrow \infty$, $PA_{O_2} \twoheadrightarrow PI_{O_2}$; as $\dot{V}A \twoheadrightarrow 0$, $PA_{O_2}$ moves away from $PI_{O_2}$ (or, $\twoheadrightarrow 0$). Also, qualitatively, it should be apparent that metabolic rate must be important in determining $PA_{O_2}$. That is, it is the ratio between the metabolic consumption of $O_2$ and the alveolar ventilation that should help to determine $PA_{O_2}$, just as the similar ratio ($\dot{V}CO_2/\dot{V}A$) is important in determining $PA_{CO_2}$.

The quantitative prediction of $PA_{O_2}$ is more complex than it is for $PA_{CO_2}$ for two reasons: (a) The inspired $PO_2$ ($PI_{O_2}$) is not zero; and (b) the R.Q. and therefore the respiratory exchange ratio (R) are usually less than 1.0, so that more molecules of $O_2$ are being removed from the alveolar gas per unit time than are being replaced by $CO_2$ molecules. Thus, $P_{A_{N_2}} > P_{I_{N_2}}$ simply because the molecules diluting $N_2$ ($O_2$, $CO_2$, $H_2O$) are becoming fewer in number, and the total gas pressure must stay equal to barometric pressure. The mean alveolar $P_{O_2}$ can be calculated from the following equation, called the "alveolar gas equation":

$$P_{A_{O_2}} = P_{I_{O_2}} - P_{A_{CO_2}} \left[ F_{I_{O_2}} + \frac{1 - F_{I_{O_2}}}{R} \right]$$

where $F_{I_{O_2}}$ is the fraction of $O_2$ molecules in the dry gas, $P_{I_{O_2}}$ is the inspired $P_{O_2}$ and can be calculated from $F_{I_{O_2}}$ ($P_B - P_{H_2O}$), and R is the respiratory exchange ratio, which is equal to the flow of $CO_2$ molecules across the alveolar membranes per minute divided by the flow of $O_2$ molecules across those membranes per minute ($\dot{V}_{CO_2}/\dot{V}_{O_2}$). R.Q., remember, is the ratio of $\dot{V}_{CO_2}/\dot{V}_{O_2}$ actually being produced and consumed by body metabolism per unit time. In the truly steady state, R must equal R.Q., but they may be markedly different in nonsteady states, such as the initial transients of hyperventilation and hypoventilation where body stores of $CO_2$ are being emptied or filled. So, in a normal resting man breathing room air at sea level, whose $P_{A_{CO_2}}$ is 40 mm Hg, and whose R is 0.82 (a normal value), the calculation would proceed thus:

$$P_{A_{O_2}} = 149 \text{ mm Hg} - 40 \text{ mm Hg} \left[ 0.21 + \frac{1 - 0.21}{0.82} \right]$$
$$= 149 \text{ mm Hg} - 40 \text{ mm Hg} \quad (1.17)$$

Or

$$P_{A_{O_2}} = 149 \text{ mm Hg} - 47 \text{ mm Hg} = 102 \text{ mm Hg}.$$

Again, this is a normal figure.

So, it is easily possible to get answers using this complex-looking equation. But, the equation is really more simple than it looks. Let's consider some limiting cases. For instance, if we assume the R is equal to 1.0 (the subject is metabolizing pure carbohydrate), then the expression in brackets reduces to 1.0 itself. Under these circumstances, the equation reduces to $P_{A_{O_2}} = P_{I_{O_2}} - P_{A_{CO_2}}$, or $P_{I_{O_2}} = P_{A_{O_2}} + P_{A_{CO_2}}$, or $P_{I_{O_2}} - P_{A_{O_2}} = P_{A_{CO_2}}$. In other words, if one molecule of $O_2$ moves from alveolar gas to blood for each molecule of $CO_2$ that moves from blood to alveolar gas, then $P_{A_{O_2}}$ will be lower than $P_{I_{O_2}}$ by an amount exactly equal to the amount by which $P_{A_{CO_2}}$ is higher than $P_{I_{CO_2}}$ (which is normally zero or close to it). In fact, a little experimentation will convince the reader that the figure in brackets can vary only between 1.3 and 1.0 as R varies between its possible limits of 0.7 (metabolizing pure fat) and 1.0 (metabolizing pure carbohydrate). Under normal circumstances, R is between these outside limits, somewhere about 0.8–0.85, and the factor in brackets is about 1.2, as in the sample calculation above. Likewise, changing $F_{IO_2}$, for any given R, changes the factor in brackets relatively little. If one lowers the percentage of $O_2$ from its normal value of 21% down to 10%, the factor changes from 1.17 to 1.20 (R staying at 0.82). If one gives the subject pure $O_2$ to breathe, then the factor in brackets becomes 1.0 regardless of the value of R. Under these circumstances, the only gases in the alveoli are $O_2$, $H_2O$, and $CO_2$, whose total partial pressures must add up to PB. If PB = 760 mm Hg, then $P_{IO_2}$ = (760 − 47) mm Hg and $P_{AO_2}$ will be equal to (760 − 47 − $P_{ACO_2}$), or $P_{IO_2}$ − $P_{ACO_2}$. It is well to realize at this juncture that PB also may change—by 10 or 20 mm Hg at any given location with changes in weather, by many hundreds of mm Hg when one ascends to high altitude, or by thousands of mm Hg if one descends to depths beneath the water or is put into a pressure chamber.

## AN EXAMPLE OF "REAL LIFE" USAGE OF THESE TWO EQUATIONS

The "alveolar gas equation," especially when used with the equation predicting $P_{ACO_2}$, can be extremely useful clinically. For example, suppose a paralyzed patient being respired by a mechanical ventilator needs to fly across the country for some reason. You wish to know if the change in pressurization will necessitate supplying $O_2$ to the patient's inspired gas, and you know that the particular aircraft involved (a DC-10) doesn't let cabin pressure fall below 573 mm Hg (equivalent to 7,600 ft.) even when flying at its maximum altitude of 42,000 ft. Suppose the respirator is adjusted at sea level to keep the patient's $P_{ACO_2}$ at 35 mm Hg, and that the patient's R = 0.80. Firstly, what will his $P_{AO_2}$ be when breathing room air at sea level?

$$P_{AO_2} = P_{IO_2} - P_{ACO_2}\left[F_{IO_2} + \frac{1 - F_{IO_2}}{R}\right]$$

$$P_{AO_2} = 149 \text{ mm Hg} - 35 \ (1.20) = 149 - 42 = 107 \text{ mm Hg.}$$

Secondly, you would want to know what would happen to his $P_{AO_2}$ under the expected conditions of cabin pressure at maximum altitude if you changed neither the settings of the ventilator nor the percentage of $O_2$ of the inspired gas. It might be that no intervention were needed, if his $P_{AO_2}$ could be expected to stay high enough to maintain adequate oxygenation and keep the patient comfortable (above 60–65 mm Hg). $P_{AO_2}$ = (573 mm Hg − 47 mm Hg) (0.21) − 42 mm Hg = 110.1 mm Hg − 42 mm Hg = 68.1 mm Hg. So, it would appear that the patient will need no intervention even at the maximum altitude that the plane is likely to reach, provided that the cabin pressurization remains operative. Now getting into the spirit of things, you decide to find out whether 100% $O_2$ would be sufficient to keep this patient oxygenated and comfortable in the unlikely event of a loss of pressurization at 42,000 ft. (PB = 128 mm Hg).

$$\text{PA}_{O_2} = (128 - 47) - 35 = 46 \text{ mm Hg}$$

Well, that may not be high enough for comfort, although the patient would be expected to stay conscious and reasonably alert, and obviously the pilot would waste little time getting down to a lower altitude. While up at 42,000 ft., however, you could improve matters considerably for the patient by increasing his alveolar ventilation (as the regulatory mechanisms of most of the normal passengers will do). Suppose you increase his $\dot{V}A$ to seven-fifths of what it was, thereby decreasing his $\text{PA}_{CO_2}$ to five-sevenths of what it was. The new $\text{PA}_{CO_2}$ will be, in the steady state, 25 mm Hg; and the new $\text{PA}_{O_2}$, at 42,000 ft., depressurized, and with the patient breathing pure $O_2$, will be 56 mm Hg. Now, a rise of 10 mm Hg in $\text{PA}_{O_2}$ may not seem like much, but it makes a world of difference in the arterial blood oxygen content. The subject of $O_2$ carriage in blood is dealt with in detail in the next chapter, and the interested reader is directed there for in-depth information. Let me just say here that the arterial hemoglobin would be about 75% saturated at a $\text{PA}_{O_2}$ of 46 and would be about 88% saturated at a $\text{PA}_{O_2}$ of 56. Most people would feel very much more comfortable under the latter conditions than they would under the former.

## REFERENCES: SUGGESTED READINGS

1. Comroe, Julius H., Jr. (1974): *Physiology of Respiration.* Year Book Medical Publishers, Chicago.
2. Otis, Arthur B. (1964): Quantitative relationships in steady-state gas exchange. In: *Handbook of Physiology, Sect. 3: Respiration,* edited by W. O. Fenn and H. Rahn, Vol. 1. American Physiological Society, Washington, D.C.

## PROBLEMS

1. The following measurements were obtained from a basal subject in the steady state breathing air in Bishop, California. Use them to answer A–G.

| | |
|---|---|
| $V_T$ | 500 ml, BTPS |
| $V_D$ | 140 ml, BTPS |
| f | 15 breaths/min |
| $\text{PA}_{CO_2}$ | 35 mm Hg |
| $P_B$ | 650 mm Hg |
| $P_{H_2O}$ @ 37° | 47 mm Hg |
| Body temp. | 37°C |
| Arterial pH | 7.42 |

$$\text{PA}_{O_2} = \text{FI}_{O_2}(P_B - 47) - \text{PA}_{CO_2}\left[\text{FI}_{O_2} + \frac{1 - \text{FI}_{O_2}}{R}\right]$$

A. From the above data, calculate the subject's alveolar ventilation: $\dot{V}A =$ _____ liters/min, BTPS

B. From the above data, calculate the subject's carbon dioxide production:
$\dot{V}CO_2 = $ _____liters/min, STPD

C. Assuming the subject increases his respiratory frequency voluntarily by one-third without changing his tidal volume, what will be the new steady-state $CO_2$?
$PA_{CO_2} = $ _____mm Hg

D. Assuming instead that the subject increases his tidal volume by one-third (to 667 ml) while keeping his respiratory frequency at 15 breaths/min, what will be the new alveolar $CO_2$? If this differs from your answer in C, explain why.
$PA_{CO_2}$ _____mm Hg

E. Calculate a probable value for the subject's oxygen consumption.
$\dot{V}O_2 = $ _____ml/min, STPD

F. Calculate a probable value for the subject's alveolar oxygen pressure:
$PA_{O_2} = $ _____mm Hg

G. What alveolar ventilation would this subject have to achieve to bring his alveolar oxygen pressure in Bishop, California up to the value normally expected at sea level ($P_B = 760$ mm Hg) if his metabolism did not change?
$\dot{V}A = $ _____liters/min, BTPS

2. A normal child running on a treadmill has the following data measured simultaneously in the steady state: Use them to answer questions A–C.

| | |
|---|---|
| $V_T$ | 800 ml, BTPS |
| $f$ | 16 breaths/min |
| Body temp. | 39°C (note that this is not 37°C.) |
| $P_{H_2O}$ at 39° | 52 mm Hg |
| Caloric equivalent of $O_2$ | 4.8 kcal/liter |
| $P_B$ | 720 mm Hg |
| $FI_{O_2}$ | 0.210 |
| $FE_{O_2}$ | 0.170 |
| $FI_{CO_2}$ | 0.000 |
| $FE_{CO_2}$ | 0.040 |
| $Pa_{CO_2}$ | 32 mm Hg |

A. His respiratory minute volume is _____liters/min
B. His physiological dead space is _____ml/breath
C. His alveolar $P_{CO_2}$ is _____mm Hg

3. A subject is breathing with a tidal volume of 0.5 liters, a dead space of 0.15 liter and a frequency of 10 breaths/min, so that his total minute volume

is 5 liters/min. He then changes his breathing pattern to a tidal volume of 0.3 liter, a frequency of 20/min, and a total minute volume of 6 liters/min. Assuming no change in dead space, this would affect alveolar ventilation as follows:

a. increase by 1 liter/min
b. increase by 0.5 liter/min
c. no change
d. decrease by 0.5 liter/min
e. decrease by 1 liter/min

4. The record in Fig. 5 represents the results of giving a patient a single breath of 100% oxygen to inspire. From that record, his anatomical dead space is closest to

a. 100 ml
b. 150 ml
c. 200 ml
d. 450 ml
e. 550 ml

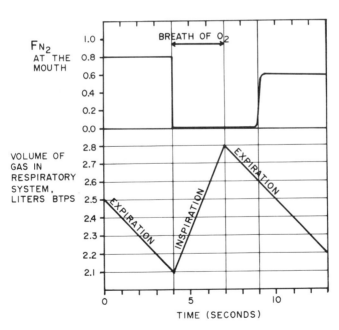

**FIG. 5.** Airway $FN_2$ and volume of air in the respiratory system both vs time as a patient is given a single breath of 100% $O_2$.

## ANSWERS

1. **A:** $\dot{V}_A = f(V_T - V_D) = 15(500 - 150) = 5{,}250$ ml/min, BTPS.
   **B:** $P_{ACO_2} = 863$ mm Hg $(\dot{V}_{CO_2}$, STPD$)/\dot{V}_A$, BTPS$)$. Rearranging:

$$\dot{V}_{CO_2, \text{STPD}} = \frac{P_{ACO_2}(\dot{V}_A, \text{BTPS})}{863 \text{ mm Hg}} = \frac{35 \text{ mm Hg } (5{,}250 \text{ ml/min})}{863 \text{ mm Hg}}$$

$$= 213 \text{ ml/min, STPD}$$

**C:** From the equation in **A** above, $\dot{V}_A$ is directly proportional to respiratory frequency. From the equation in **B**, $P_{ACO_2}$ is inversely proportional to $\dot{V}_A$. Thus, $P_{ACO_2}$ must be inversely proportional to respiratory frequency here, since the tidal volume and metabolic rate are constant in this steady state. So, if it is increased to become four-thirds of what it was, $P_{ACO_2}$ must become three-fourths of what it was in the new steady state: $3/4(35 \text{ mm Hg}) = 26$ mm Hg.

**D:** Using the equation in **A**, $\dot{V}_A = 15(667 - 150) = 7{,}755$ ml/min, BTPS. Using the equation in **B** along with the $\dot{V}_{CO_2}$ calculated in **B**, we get

$$P_{ACO_2} = 863 \text{ mm Hg} \frac{213 \text{ ml/min, STPD}}{7{,}755 \text{ ml/min, BTPS}} = 24 \text{ mm Hg}$$

Note that this is lower than the answer to **C** because increased $V_T$, unlike increased f, does not increase $f(V_D)$.

**E:** Since the subject is basal, $R \approx 0.82$. $R = \dot{V}_{CO_2}/\dot{V}_{O_2}$, and $\dot{V}_{O_2} = \dot{V}_{CO_2}/R$. Using the $\dot{V}_{CO_2}$ found in **B**, $\dot{V}_{O_2} = 213/0.82 = 260$ ml/min, STPD.
**F:** Using the alveolar gas equation and remembering that dry air is about 21% $O_2$

$$P_{AO_2} = 0.21(650 - 47) - 35\left[0.21 + \frac{1-0.21}{0.82}\right] = 86 \text{ mm Hg}$$

**G:** This is a devious calculation, even considering the physiologists' diabolical bent of mind! Begin by calculating a normal sea-level $P_{AO_2}$, remembering that, at sea level, the normal $P_{ACO_2}$ is 40, not 35:

$$P_{AO_2} = 0.21(760 - 47) - 40\left[0.21 + \frac{0.79}{0.82}\right] = 103.$$

Substitute this in the value for Bishop and solve for $P_{ACO_2}$ there:

$$103 \text{ mm Hg} = 0.21(650 - 47) - P_{ACO_2}\left[0.21 + \frac{0.79}{0.82}\right]$$

$$P_{ACO_2} = 20 \text{ mm Hg}$$

If $P_{ACO_2}$ has decreased to four-sevenths of what it was $(20/35)$, then $\dot{V}_A$ must be seven-fourths what it was. So, $(7/4)(5250 \text{ ml/min}) = 9{,}188$ ml/min, BTPS.

2. **A:** 0.8 liter/breath (16 breaths/min) = 12.8 liters/min.

   **B:** $PE_{CO_2} = FE_{CO_2}(PB - PH_2O) = 0.04 (720 - 52) = 26.7$ mm Hg. Since the child is normal, we can assume that $PA_{CO_2} = Pa_{CO_2} = 32$ mm Hg, and we can use the Bohr formula: $VD = VT(PA_{CO_2} - PE_{CO_2})/PA_{CO_2} = 132$ ml/breath.

   **C:** As just stated, $PA_{CO_2}$ must be equal to $Pa_{CO_2}$, or 32 mm Hg.

3. In the first case, $\dot{V}A = (0.5 - 0.15)10 = 3.5$ liters/min, BTPS. In the second case, $\dot{V}A = (0.3 - 0.15)20 = 3.0$ liters/min, BTPS. Thus, the answer (d).

4. The subject begins to expire at the 7-second mark. From there until the line "squaring of" the rise of $FN_2$ (at the 9-second mark), exactly 200 ml of gas have flowed out of the respiratory system. Thus, the anatomical dead space is 200 ml, or answer (c).

# 4

# *Oxygen Carriage by Blood*

In the previous chapter the usage of the alveolar gas equation to predict $P_{A_{O_2}}$ was discussed in some detail. That $P_{A_{O_2}}$ then serves as a pressure source. In the lungs, one "connects" this pressure source simultaneously to two very different-sized $O_2$ reservoirs. These reservoirs, which had emptied somewhat at the tissues, proceed to "fill up" until their pressures are essentially equal to that of the source. Thus, if exchange were ideal, the arterial blood could be said to have the same partial pressure as that of the alveolar gas. The amount of $O_2$ transferred from the source per minute to the two reservoirs depends on three factors: (a) How much blood containing these reservoirs is "connected" to the source each minute, (b) How empty the reservoirs are on their arrival (how much $O_2$ has been used by the tissues), and (c) How fully the reservoirs are filled, which depends primarily on $P_{A_{O_2}}$. These factors are quantitatively related to one another in Fick's equation ($\dot{V}_{O_2} = \dot{Q}(Ca_{O_2} - C\bar{v}_{O_2})$). In this chapter I would like to consider the characteristics of the two reservoirs in which $O_2$ is carried in blood. Oxygen is carried (a) physically dissolved, and (b) chemically bound to hemoglobin (Hb).

## OXYGEN IN PHYSICAL SOLUTION

The oxygen physically dissolved in blood follows Henry's law, which states that the amount of gas dissolved is directly proportional to the partial pressure with which the liquid is in equilibrium. Stated symbolically, $[O_2]_{diss} = \alpha(P_{O_2})$, where $\alpha$ for $O_2$ dissolved in blood is $(0.03$ ml $O_2/\text{liter})/\text{mm Hg}$. Thus, if the arterial $P_{O_2}$ ($Pa_{O_2}$) is 100 mm Hg, there are 3 ml $O_2$ dissolved in each liter of that blood.

Three milliliters of $O_2$ isn't much when compared with the oxygen consumption of a resting person. If the dissolved reservoir were the only one, then an astonishing flow of blood would be required simply to supply the tissues with their resting oxygen consumption ($\dot{V}_{O_2}$). Assuming that the resting $\dot{V}_{O_2}$ is 250 ml/min, and that all of the dissolved reservoir of $O_2$ is available to the tissues, Fick's equation can show that the cardiac output would have to be an impossible 83.3 liters/min under these circumstances.

If a subject breathes pure $O_2$ at sea level, his $PA_{O_2}$ may rise to above 650 mm Hg, and his $Pa_{O_2}$ may be 650 mm Hg. Even under these conditions, the 19.5 ml of $O_2$ dissolved in each liter of blood still is only about 10% of the amount of $O_2$ normally carried, and the cardiovascular system would be hard pressed to deliver even the resting tissues' $\dot{V}_{O_2}$. Further, pure $O_2$ cannot be breathed at sea-level pressures for much longer than about a day without leading to lung damage because of its toxicity. For brief periods of time, however, people can breathe pure $O_2$ under pressures of greater than 1 atm. It would take pure $O_2$, under a pressure of about 10 atm, to dissolve as much $O_2$ in blood as is normally carried in both reservoirs. At these pressures, $O_2$ toxicity would cause convulsions in 1 or 2 minutes, and death shortly thereafter.

## OXYGEN BOUND TO Hb

There are about 147 g of Hb in each liter of normal blood, which calculates to a solution that is 0.00228 M in Hb. Each macromolecule of Hb consists of four subunit chains each containing an $Fe^{2+}$ ion that can bind 1 molecule of $O_2$. Thus, each liter of blood should be able to carry 0.00912 M of $O_2$ if all of the binding sites were filled, or 204 ml $O_2$/liter of blood. In fact, the $O_2$ capacity of 147 g of Hb is only about 197 ml $O_2$ (which amounts to 1.34 ml $O_2$/g Hb), a figure in common usage. Presumably this small disparity exists because some small percentage of the Hb molecules are incapable of binding to $O_2$, perhaps as a result of their normal $Fe^{2+}$ ion having been oxidized to $Fe^{3+}$ (methemoglobin). Carbon monoxide may also contribute to this disparity, since it binds to Hb far more strongly than does $O_2$ (210 times as strongly) and therefore may make some sites unavailable for $O_2$ binding.

The relationship between the amount of $O_2$ bound to Hb [actually, the ordinate is percent saturation of Hb = $\{[HbO_2]/[HbO_2]_{max}\}100$] and the partial pressure of $O_2$ with which the Hb is in equilibrium is the complex sigmoid one seen in Fig. 1. Important as a determinant of this curve's shape is the fact that the four individual binding sites on a given Hb molecule interact with one another: When the first site has bound a molecule of $O_2$, the binding of the next site is facilitated; the binding of $O_2$ to the next site facilitates the third, and so forth. The result is a curve that is quite steep from 0 to 40 mm Hg, rounds off from 40 to 60 mm Hg, and is fairly flat thereafter. I would call the reader's attention to the conditions under which this curve and the tabular data with it were obtained: In normal adult man, blood pH = 7.4, body temperature = 37°C, [Hb] = 147 g/liter. Changing these variables changes the data.

## "ASSOCIATION" PART OF CURVE

The flat part of the curve (at sea level) might be called the "lung" or association part because $PA_{O_2}$ at sea level is maintained around 100 mm Hg. If the blood

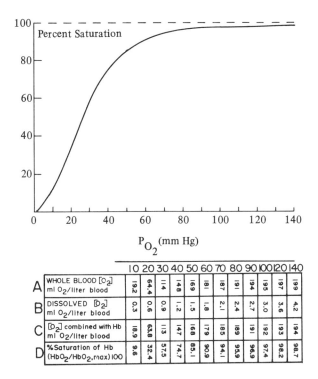

| | | 10 | 20 | 30 | 40 | 50 | 60 | 70 | 80 | 90 | 100 | 120 | 140 |
|---|---|---|---|---|---|---|---|---|---|---|---|---|---|
| A | WHOLE BLOOD [O₂] ml O₂/liter blood | 19.2 | 64.4 | 11.4 | 14.8 | 16.9 | 18.1 | 18.7 | 19.1 | 19.4 | 19.5 | 19.7 | 19.9 |
| B | DISSOLVED [O₂] ml O₂/liter blood | 0.3 | 0.6 | 0.9 | 1.2 | 1.5 | 1.8 | 2.1 | 2.4 | 2.7 | 3.0 | 3.6 | 4.2 |
| C | [O₂] combined with Hb ml O₂/liter blood | 18.9 | 63.8 | 113 | 147 | 168 | 179 | 185 | 189 | 191 | 192 | 193 | 194 |
| D | %Saturation of Hb (HbO₂/HbO₂,max)100 | 9.6 | 32.4 | 57.5 | 74.7 | 85.1 | 90.9 | 94.1 | 95.9 | 96.9 | 97.4 | 98.2 | 98.7 |

**FIG. 1.** Standard HbO₂ dissociation curve in graphical and tabular form. Normal man, HbA, pH = 7.4, body temperature (37°C), [Hb] = 147 g/liter blood. (Data of J. W. Severinghaus: *J. Appl. Physiol.*, 46:599, 1979.)

going through the lungs comes into equilibrium with a Po₂ near that, enough O₂ will be loaded onto the Hb reservoir to result in 97.4% saturation of the potential Hb binding sites. Because the curve is so flat above and below that Po₂, however, the amount of O₂ loaded onto the Hb stays roughly constant even when PA_{O_2} varies by ±20 mm Hg. That is, if PA_{O_2} were only 80 mm Hg, Hb would still be 95.9% saturated, and PA_{O_2} could rise to 120 mm Hg with Hb being only slightly more saturated (98.2%). PA_{O_2} would have to drop below 60 mm Hg for Hb saturation to drop near 90%! The "take-home" message is that the flat part of the curve assures that roughly the same amount of O₂ will be loaded onto the Hb in the lungs even if PA_{O_2} is caused to change somewhat.

## "DISSOCIATION" PART OF CURVE

The part of the curve below 60 mm Hg might be called the "tissue" or dissociation part. In the tissues, Hb must release amounts of oxygen sufficient to maintain metabolism, at partial pressures sufficiently high to drive the O₂ between capillaries and mitochondria. Since mitochondrial Po₂ may get as low as 1–3 mm Hg, the driving pressure available to cause $O_2$ to diffuse is essentially equal to the mean capillary $Po_2$ ($P\bar{c}_{o_2}$). Thus, if more $O_2$ can be released from Hb while keeping the $P\bar{c}_{o_2}$ reasonably high, more $O_2$ can be supplied per unit time to the tissues. Figure 1 shows that although less than 10% of the $O_2$ is released from Hb as $Po_2$ drops 40 mm Hg, from 100 to 60 mm Hg, almost 60% is released as $Po_2$ falls another 40 mm Hg, from 60 to 20 mm Hg. Of course, rapidly metabolizing tissues cause the Hb reservoir to empty more fully because they expose the capillary blood to lower $Po_2$ as it passes through them. This is an extremely important mechanism which operates automatically in matching tissue oxygen supply to tissue oxygen need.

But the Hb–$O_2$ dissociation curve is even better adapted to supply tissues with $O_2$. Remember that the data in Fig. 1 were obtained at pH 7.4 and temperature 37°C. Either increased temperature or increased acidity (decreased pH) tend to shift the curve to the right, as seen in Fig. 2A,B. The effect of acid on the curve is called the Bohr shift. Working tissues are both hotter and more acid than arterial blood; this is because two of the products of metabolism are heat and acids, mostly $CO_2$, which hydrates to form $H_2CO_3$, which in turn dissociates into $H^+$ and $HCO_3^-$. ($CO_2$ itself probably shifts the curve to the right independent of its ability to form $H^+$ ions.) The more intense a given tissue's metabolism is, the more its temperature and acidity will be elevated, thus shifting the Hb-$O_2$ curve of blood brought to it further and further to the right. The curve's shifting to the right allows the mean capillary $Po_2$ to be kept high even as working tissues remove more of the $O_2$ from the Hb.

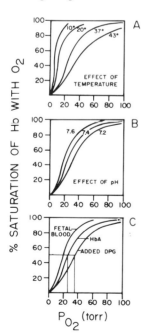

FIG. 2. Variations in the Hb-$O_2$ dissociation curve. **A:** Effect of changes in temperature; **B:** Effect of changes in blood pH; **C:** Hyperbolic curve of "purified" HbA (dialyzed to be salt-free) is similar to curve of myoglobin (Mb); **D:** The dissociation curve of fetal blood (but not pure HbF) is to the left of adult blood containing HbA; addition of DPG shifts curve of blood with HbA to the right and increases $P_{50}$ (decreases affinity of $O_2$ for Hb and facilitates unloading of $O_2$ in tissues). (Reproduced with permission from Comroe, J. H., Jr.: *Physiology of Respiration,* 2nd Ed. Copyright © 1974 by Year Book Medical Publishers, Chicago.)

These mechanisms thus stabilize the mean capillary $P_{O_2}$, and therefore the tissue $P_{O_2}$, in the face of variable $O_2$ demand by the tissues. It should be pointed out here that both temperature and acidity also affect loading of $O_2$ in the lungs, but the effect is very small for several reasons: (a) In the lungs the $P_{CO_2}$ and acidity are brought back down by $CO_2$ exchange. (b) Both the normal (pH = 7.4, T = 37°C) and the hotter, more acid blood have Hb-$O_2$ dissociation curves which flatten out, reaching near 100% saturation at normal $P_{A_{O_2}}$.

## 2,3-DIPHOSPHOGLYCERATE

Another substance that profoundly affects the tissue or dissociation part of the Hb-$O_2$ dissociation curve is 2,3-diphosphoglycerate (2,3-DPG). It is present in much higher concentrations in red cells (15 mm/g Hb) than in other cells because the red cells utilize a shunt that converts much of their 1,3-DPG to 2,3-DPG. Figure 3 shows the glycolytic pathway in most cells (the vertical pathway from glucose through pyruvate and lactate). It also shows the shunt pathway by which red cells convert much of their 1,3-DPG to 2,3-DPG through the action of DPG mutase. 2,3-DPG, like $H^+$ ions, is bound much more strongly by deoxygenated Hb than by oxygenated Hb.

Figure 2C compares the Hb dissociation curves of normal fetal blood, (but not pure HbF), normal adult blood (containing HbA), and normal adult blood with added 2,3-DPG, which has the lowest affinity for $O_2$ (shown furthest to

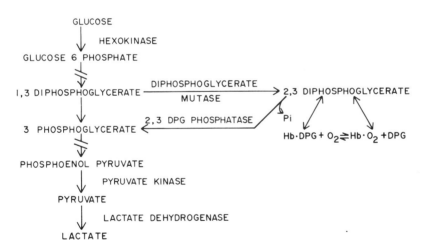

**FIG. 3.** Formation of 2,3-DPG in erythrocytes. The vertical chain at the left shows the glycolytic pathway in cells other than erythrocytes. In erythrocytes, the enzyme DPG mutase catalyzes the conversion of much of the 1,3-DPG to 2,3-DPG. That not bound by deoxygenated Hb is converted to 3-phosphoglycerate without the formation of adenosine triphosphate. The enzyme catalyzing the formation of 2,3-DPG is strongly inhibited by free 2,3-DPG; thus the level of free 2,3-DPG can control its own production, i.e., when more DPG is bound by deoxygenated Hb, the concentration of DPG decreases and its formation is increased.

the right). Quantitatively, the values of $Po_2$ at which the Hb of the three bloods would be half-saturated with $O_2$ are respectively, 19, 26, and 37 mm Hg. Interestingly enough, pure HbA, whose four subunits are two $\alpha$- and two $\beta$-chains, has slightly more $O_2$ affinity than pure HbF (i.e., HbA lies to the left of pure HbF), which consists of two $\alpha$- and two $\gamma$-chains. The reversal of this hierarchy in normal fetal and adult blood seems entirely due to the former not binding 2,3-DPG as strongly as the latter; thus adult blood is pushed far to the right of fetal blood at normal concentrations of 2,3-DPG, and even further to the right at still higher concentrations of 2,3-DPG. It is fortunate that fetal blood has such a high affinity for $O_2$, for the $Po_2$ of fetal blood as it leaves the placenta on its way back to the fetus is only about 30 mm Hg. Normal adult blood would only be about 55% saturated at this $Po_2$, but fetal blood is about 75% saturated.

Since the level of 2,3-DPG is so instrumental in determining the $O_2$ affinity of blood, it becomes important to consider what factors may control the rate of formation of 2,3-DPG. *Firstly,* the formation of 2,3-DPG is inhibited by high concentrations of free 2,3-DPG. If more 2,3-DPG is bound because there is more deoxygenated Hb present (as might occur during exposure to an environment low in $O_2$), the level of free 2,3-DPG is decreased, leading to an increase in its formation. *Secondly,* alkalosis stimulates glycolysis in general and may lead to increased rates of formation of 2,3-DPG. *Thirdly,* there is some evidence that hormones such as thyroxin, testosterone, growth hormone, and catecholamines may exert an effect on $O_2$ affinity through an effect on 2,3-DPG metabolism.

Let us now consider a few examples that illustrate the role of 2,3-DPG as a regulator of oxygen transport to tissues.

1. *Storage of blood in banks.* The level of 2,3-DPG decreases during storage, becoming quite low within about a week. This blood will have an Hb-$O_2$ dissociation curve far to the left, making it difficult for tissues to obtain $O_2$. Since it may take 6–24 hours for the 2,3-DPG levels to approach normal, care should be exercised in the use of this blood in sick patients, especially those likely to need many units of it. Thus, a patient scheduled for open heart surgery, which requires multiple units of blood during cardiopulmonary bypass, might be a very poor risk if bank blood is used.

2. *Treatment of patients with chronic metabolic acidosis.* The acute effects of the acidosis would be to push the Hb-$O_2$ curve to the right, and (by inhibiting glycolysis) to decrease the rate of formation of 2,3-DPG. In time, therefore, the decreased rate of formation of the 2,3-DPG would return the Hb-$O_2$ curve back toward normal even in the presence of acidosis. In a severely acidotic patient, the physician may wish to help the kidneys restore the patient's acid–base status by infusing a solution of $NaHCO_3$. Care must be exercised! The reduction of the acidosis will directly shift the Hb-$O_2$ curve to the left (making it harder for the tissues to obtain $O_2$). Of course, it will also increase the rate

of formation of 2,3-DPG and tend to restore the curve back toward normal. Again, the readjustment of levels of 2,3-DPG takes time (6–24 hours), and the correction of the acid–base state should be done slowly.

3. *Residence at high altitude.* Acute exposure to an environment low in $O_2$ leads to increased breathing and therefore decreased $P_{CO_2}$ and alkalosis. The alkalosis is accentuated in the red blood cells because deoxygenated Hb binds $H^+$ more avidly. Thus, the Hb-$O_2$ curve is shifted to the left acutely, and, at a time when loading of $O_2$ at the lungs may be compromised by low $P_{AO_2}$, unloading of $O_2$ at the tissues is also compromised by the alkalosis. Fortunately, the increased amount of deoxygenated Hb binds 2,3-DPG more avidly, decreasing its free concentration, and the alkalosis stimulates glycolysis. Both factors tend to increase formation of 2,3-DPG and restore the position of the Hb-$O_2$ curve back toward normal with the usual time course.

## CARBON MONOXIDE

Carbon monoxide combines with Hb at the same site at which oxygen does, but its bond is 210 times as strong as that of oxygen. Thus, if a sample of blood were *equilibrated* with normal air (21% $O_2$) contaminated with just 0.1% CO, half the binding sites would be occupied with $O_2$ and half with CO. The $F_{AO_2}$ is normally not 0.21 but rather about 0.14 ($P_{AO_2}$ about 100 mm Hg); if the pulmonary blood flow were to equilibrate with normal alveolar gas contaminated with only 0.066% CO, the Hb binding sites would be half occupied by CO and half occupied by $O_2$. Fortunately for smokers and those of us who must travel through tunnels, the inhalation of 0.1% CO doesn't quickly lead to 50% HbCO because so little CO is breathed in per unit time. We can quickly calculate that a person who inspires 6 liters/min of gas at that percentage of CO inspires 6 ml of CO/min. This normal person has about 6 liters of blood, each liter of which can combine with 200 ml of CO. At *half*-saturation with CO, therefore, his blood volume will hold 600 ml CO, and he will have to breathe 0.1% CO for 100 min just to take in that much.

An otherwise normal person whose arterial blood was 50% HbCO and 50% HbO₂ would be collapsed or on the verge of collapse, while a person who was normal except for a Hb concentration only half of normal (and therefore who also had half the normal content of $O_2$ per liter of arterial blood) can function normally at rest and may even have a considerable exercise tolerance. Carbon monoxide does more than just lower the $O_2$ content of arterial blood; it shifts the Hb-$O_2$ dissociation curve to the left and makes release of $O_2$ to the tissues extremely difficult. Figure 4 contrasts the Hb-$O_2$ dissociation curves of normal blood, anemic blood, and blood that is normal except for having 20, 40, or 60% of its Hb bound to CO. The curve is plotted on a graph whose ordinate is $O_2$ content, rather than percent saturation as has been used in Figs. 1 and 2. The curves of the normal blood and the anemic blood have exactly the same shape, the anemic blood holding exactly four-tenths as much $O_2$ as

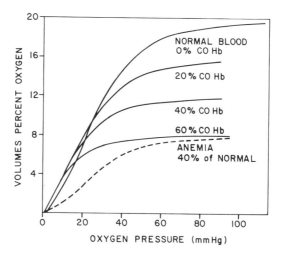

**FIG. 4.** Oxygen dissociation curves of human blood at pH 7.4 and 38°C, containing various percentages of carboxyhemoglobin *(solid lines)*, and of anemic human blood containing only 40% of the normal Hb content *(dotted line)*. (Reproduced with permission from Roughton, F. J. W., Transport of oxygen and carbon dioxide. In: *Handbook of Physiology, Sect. 3: Respiration,* edited by W. O. Fenn and H. Rahn, Vol. 1. Washington, D.C., American Physiological Society, 1964.)

the normal blood at any given $P_{O_2}$. The curves of the 20, 40, and 60% HbCO bloods are all shifted to the left of the normal, and there is a really startling separation between the anemia curve and the 60% HbCO curve, although both hold equal amounts of $O_2$/liter at a normal arterial $P_{O_2}$ of about 100 mm Hg. Lowering the blood $P_{O_2}$ to 20 mm Hg will cause the anemic blood to release 70% of its $O_2$ to the tissues; lowering the 60% HbCO blood $P_{O_2}$ to 20 mm Hg will release only about 25% of its $O_2$ to the tissues. This degree of CO poisoning (60% HbCO) might well be fatal.

Carbon monoxide is particularly dangerous because it is so insidious. It is colorless, tasteless, odorless, nonirritating; it causes no increase in ventilation, no sensation of breathlessness, and no cyanosis (because the color of HbCO is cherry red). Thus, an individual can breathe lethal concentrations of CO until enough of his Hb is bound to CO to cause collapse, without ever being aware of the danger.

## REFERENCES

1. Comroe, J. H., Jr. (1974): *Physiology of Respiration,* 2nd Ed., p. 316. Year Book Medical Publishers, Chicago.
2. Control mechanisms for oxygen release (a series of four papers dealing with 2,3-DPG and hemoglobin) (1970): *Fed. Proc.,* 29(3):1101–117.
3. Roughton, F. J. W. (1964): Transport of oxygen and carbon dioxide. In: *Handbook of Physiology, Sect. 3, Respiration,* edited by, W. O. Fenn and H. Rahn, Vol. 1, p. 767. American Physiological Society, Washington, D.C.

**PROBLEMS**

1. An artificial blood oxygenator would be most effective in loading Hb with oxygen if it were

   a. at 20°C, pH 7.2
   b. at 20°C, pH 7.6
   c. at 37°C, pH 7.2
   d. at 37°C, pH 7.4
   e. at 39°C, pH 7.6

2. The shift in position of the Hb-$O_2$ curve that occurs acutely in a metabolic acidosis would

   a. increase the ability of Hb to take up $O_2$ in the lungs
   b. have no effect on tissue $O_2$ tension
   c. be in the same direction as that produced by decreased temperature
   d. increase the venous oxygen tension
   e. decrease the pressure at which $O_2$ is delivered to tissue cells

3. Chemical combination of $O_2$ with Hb tends to

   a. decrease the affinity of Hb for protons
   b. decrease the affinity of any other $O_2$-binding sites on the same Hb molecule for $O_2$
   c. make the blood bluer in color
   d. make the blood more alkaline
   e. form a stronger bond than that formed by Hb and CO

4. All of the following tend to shift the Hb-$O_2$ dissociation curve to the right *except*

   a. increased temperature
   b. respiratory acidosis
   c. increased DPG concentration
   d. increased CO concentration
   e. metabolic acidosis

5. On the graph in Fig. 5 are superimposed five points marked 1–5. These points represent samples of blood that could have been drawn from people under different conditions, and from different sites in the cardiovascular system, and which were then analyzed for [$O_2$] and $P_{O_2}$ and plotted. For each condition listed below (A–E), choose the corresponding blood sample. (Samples may be used more than once.)

   A. Arterial blood from a normal person breathing 31% $O_2$ during an acute exposure to a barometric pressure of 523 mm Hg.
   B. Mixed venous blood from a normal person breathing air while resting at sea level.

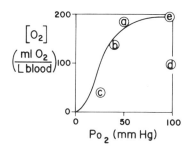

FIG. 5. This plot of $O_2$ content vs $P_{O_2}$ is derived from normal blood with an Hb concentration of 147 g/liter blood, at a pH 7.4, a $P_{CO_2}$ of 40 mm Hg, and a body temperature 37°C.

C. Arterial blood from a normal person who had arrived at 12,000 ft. an hour ago ($P_B = 483$ mm Hg), and was breathing air while resting.

D. Coronary sinus blood from a normal person during exercise at sea level breathing air.

E. Arterial blood from a person who was otherwise normal except for having been breathing air contaminated with 0.1% CO at sea level for hours.

## ANSWERS

1. Temperature and acidity shift the Hb-$O_2$ dissociation curve to the right as they increase. At any given $P_{O_2}$, therefore, an artificial blood oxygenator would load blood with the most oxygen if the blood were kept cold and alkaline. The answer is (b).

2. Acidity shifts the Hb-$O_2$ dissociation curve to the right. Clearly, then, (a) and (c) are backwards. In most tissues, the "tissue" $P_{O_2}$ is about equal to the $P_{O_2}$ in the venous blood draining that tissue; that is, the blood $P_{O_2}$ almost reaches equilibrium with the tissue so far as its $P_{O_2}$ is concerned before it leaves the tissue. So, (b), (d), and (e) are really asking whether the venous (tissue) $P_{O_2}$ stays the same, rises, or falls. If we assume that the tissues metabolize at the same rate as they normally do during the acidosis and that the blood flow to the tissues is normal, then each tissue will remove the same amount of $O_2$ from each liter of blood as it normally does, reducing the $O_2$ content to the normal venous level. Since the curve is shifted to the right, however $P_{O_2}$ will be higher than normal at normal venous $O_2$ content, and the answer is (d).

3. Both $H^+$ ions and 2,3-DPG are bound more strongly by Hb than by HbO$_2$. Thus, the answer is (a).

4. Each of the choices (a–c) and (e) *do* shift the Hb-$O_2$ curve to the right. The exception is CO, which shifts it to the left, making it difficult for the tissues to extract $O_2$ from the blood. The correct answer is (d).

5. **A:** One can calculate that the 31% $O_2$ at that low barometric pressure is sufficient to result in a normal sea-level $PI_{O_2}$. [$PI_{O_2} = FI_{O_2} (PB - 47) = 0.31 (523 - 47) = 147.5$ mm Hg.] Thus, there is no reason why $PA_{O_2}$ should not be normal, and the blood should load up with a normal amount of $O_2$ as it goes through the lungs, or nearly 200 ml $O_2$/liter blood. There is also no reason why the pH, temperature, 2,3-DPG content of the blood should be anything but normal, and so the blood sample should lie on the normal curve. The correct answer is 5.

**B:** Mixed venous blood in a person breathing room air at sea level at rest would have an $O_2$ content of about 140–150 ml $O_2$/liter corresponding to a $PO_2$ of about 40 mm Hg. It would also be more acidic than 7.4, and have a higher $PCO_2$ than 40 mm Hg, so the sample should be on a curve shifted to the right from the normal one. The best answer is therefore 2.

**C:** This normal person would have a $PI_{O_2}$ of 91.5 mm Hg, and using the alveolar gas equation [$PA_{O_2} = PI_{O_2} - PA_{CO_2}\{FI_{O_2} + (1 - FI_{O_2})/R\}$], along with reasonable assumptions for $PA_{CO_2}$ and R, one can calculate that his $PA_{O_2}$ would be about 50 mm Hg. Since this is sufficiently low to cause some hyperventilation and respiratory alkalosis in normal people, this sample would be to the left of the normal curve. The correct answer is 1.

**D:** The heart, even at rest, normally removes far more of the $O_2$ from the blood perfusing it than most other organs (about 70% compared with the overall average of only about 25%). During exercise, even more than 70% of the $O_2$ may be extracted by the heart. Also, especially during exercise, the venous blood from the myocardium will be much more acid than 7.4 and have a considerably higher $PCO_2$ than 40, and will therefore be on a curve to the right of the normal one. The correct answer is therefore 3.

**E:** A normal person at sea level would have a $PA_{O_2}$ of about 100 mm Hg. Since Hb binds to CO 210 times as avidly as it binds to $O_2$, a $PA_{CO}$ of 0.48 mm Hg corresponding to 0.07% CO, would compete equally with the $O_2$, resulting in the Hb being half $HbO_2$ and half HbCO in the arterial blood. Thus the $O_2$ content would be about half normal, or about 100 ml $O_2$/liter blood, at a $PO_2$ of 100 mm Hg. The answer is 4.

# 5

# Carriage of CO₂ by Blood

Blood brings to tissues foodstuffs, and $O_2$ with which to oxidize them; the primary products of this oxidation are $CO_2$, $H_2O$, heat, and high energy phosphate bonds. The blood then must remove from the tissues the first three of these products, which might be called the "waste products" of this process. You will remember that a normal-sized person uses about 250 ml $O_2$/min at rest, and produces about 200 ml $CO_2$/min at rest. (These numbers may go up 20 times in heavy exercise.) One can easily calculate that resting metabolism in such a person produces about 0.16 g $H_2O$/min or about 231 g $H_2O$/day, and produces about 1.22 kcal of heat/min. You will remember also that the resting cardiac output in a normal person is about 5 liters/min. It is easy to see that the addition of 0.16 ml $H_2O$ to this 5 liters of flow will not provide too much of a problem. Nor will the heat, for 1.22 kcal added each minute to the 5 liters of the cardiac output will tend to raise the temperature of the blood by only about 0.24°C, assuming that the specific heat of blood is about 1. Of course, both water and heat must be removed from the blood at the same rate at which they are being added to it if the system is to remain in the steady state.

The blood must also carry away the $CO_2$, and a production of 200 ml/min means that 40 ml must be added to each liter of blood in our normal resting person. Since $CO_2$ tends to form $H^+$ ions, the blood must have buffers to prevent large pH changes from occurring. In fact, the amount of $CO_2$ produced during a day of resting metabolism in a normal person is potentially capable of forming almost 13,000 mEq of $H^+$, an enormous acid load!

This chapter begins by considering the three forms in which $CO_2$ is carried in blood. Next is a step-by-step coverage of the particulars involved as $CO_2$ moves from tissues to blood. Finally, the $CO_2$ and $O_2$ dissociation curves are drawn on the same axes and compared, and the physiological relevance of this comparison is discussed.

## THE FORMS IN WHICH $CO_2$ IS CARRIED IN BLOOD ARE (1) PHYSICALLY DISSOLVED, (2) BOUND TO PROTEINS AS CARBAMINO COMPOUNDS, AND (3) BICARBONATE

Physically dissolved $CO_2$ follows Henry's law, as did the physically dissolved $O_2$; however, $CO_2$ is more than 20 times as soluble as $O_2$ in aqueous solutions. Thus $[CO_2]_{diss} = \alpha(P_{CO_2})$, where $\alpha$ for $CO_2$ is $(0.7$ ml $CO_2$/liter)/mm Hg $P_{CO_2}$. At a normal arterial $P_{CO_2}$ of 40 mm Hg, therefore, there would be 28 ml $CO_2$ physically dissolved in each liter of plasma. This amounts to about 5% of the total amount of $CO_2$ carried in the arterial blood.

Proteins can bind $CO_2$ reversibly to their amine groups, and there is much protein in the blood. The plasma is a 7% solution of plasma proteins, and the red cells are about 30% Hb. Thus, R-$NH_2$ + $CO_2$ $\rightleftarrows$ R-$NHCOO^-$ + $H^+$. The pK of this system, insofar as Hb is concerned, is below 6, so that almost all of the $H^+$ will be ionized at physiological pH. This means that although this mechanism is useful in carrying $CO_2$ in blood it will not prevent large pH changes, because almost every $CO_2$ molecule thus bound results in an $H^+$ ion being formed. Again, about 5% of the $CO_2$ normally carried in arterial blood is in the form of carbamino compounds.

The rest of the $CO_2$ carried in blood, about 90% of the total, is carried in the form of $HCO_3^-$ ions. They are formed through the hydration of $CO_2$ and the subsequent dissociation of $H_2CO_3$, as follows: $CO_2$ + $H_2O$ $\rightleftarrows$ $H_2CO_3$ $\rightleftarrows$ $HCO_3^-$ + $H^+$. Since the effective pK of the $CO_2:HCO_3^-$ system is 6.1, almost all of these $H^+$ ions will also need buffering, if the blood pH is not to change drastically. The hydration–dehydration reaction proceeds rather slowly without the presence of the enzyme, carbonic anydrase, although the dissociation–association reaction occurs essentially instantaneously without any catalytic help. One need only think of the length of time required for a glass of a carbonated drink to convert its $H_2CO_3$ to $CO_2$ to realize how slow the hydration–dehydration can be without catalysis.

## $CO_2$ TRANSFER FROM TISSUES TO BLOOD

Let us now refer to Fig. 1 which is a schematic representation of the processes occurring as $CO_2$ moves from the tissues through the plasma and into the red blood cells. (For a scheme of lung gas exchange, reverse the direction of all arrows.) The $CO_2$ production moves first through the various membranous barriers into the blood plasma (heavy arrow). There, some dissolves in the plasma water, some binds to the amine groups of plasma proteins to form carbamino compounds (and $H^+$ ions), and some becomes hydrated to $H_2CO_3$, which dissociates into $HCO_3^-$ and more $H^+$ ions. The $H^+$ ions that are released when the carbamino compounds and $HCO_3^-$ are formed can largely be buffered by the plasma proteins (more about buffering and acid–base balance in the next chapter).

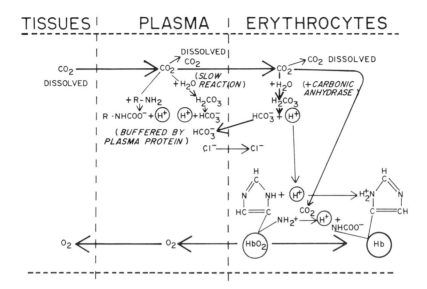

**FIG. 1.** Schematic representation of $CO_2$ passing from tissues into the plasma and into the erythrocytes as $O_2$ passes in the opposite direction. The buffering of hydrogen ions is emphasized by circling the $H^+$ that are released and buffered. (Redrawn from Davenport, H. W.: *The ABC of Acid-Base Chemistry,* 4th Ed., University of Chicago Press, Chicago, 1958.)

However, relatively little $CO_2$ gets hydrated in the plasma because there is no carbonic anhydrase to speed up the reaction there, and most of the $CO_2$ continues to diffuse through the plasma and into the red blood cells; here again, some dissolves. Some $CO_2$ forms carbamino hemoglobin with the amine groups of Hb, liberating $H^+$ ions in the process. Most of the $CO_2$ that diffuses out of the tissues, however, is fated to go through the hydration and subsequent dissociation reactions that lead to the formation of $HCO_3^-$ and $H^+$ in the red cells, because there is a plentiful supply of carbonic anhydrase to speed up the hydration. The $H^+$ ions that were released when the carbamino-Hb and $HCO_3^-$ were formed are then efficiently buffered by the ubiquitous Hb molecules (remember, the red cells are 30% Hb). Although the Hb molecules have several types of groups capable of buffering $H^+$ ions, the most important of these are the imidazole groups of the histidine residues, as shown in Fig. 2. They are quantiatively important because Hb is rich in them, and because the pK of the group is about 7.0, which is near enough to physiological pH to be useful.

Thus, most of the $CO_2$ that is taken up by blood as it passes through tissue is converted to $HCO_3^-$ and $H^+$ ions in the red cells. This reaction is able to proceed without the products accumulating and stopping it because (a) $H^+$ ions are efficiently "mopped up" by Hb, and (b) $HCO_3^-$ ions move from red cells to plasma as their concentration in the red cells begins to increase. Most

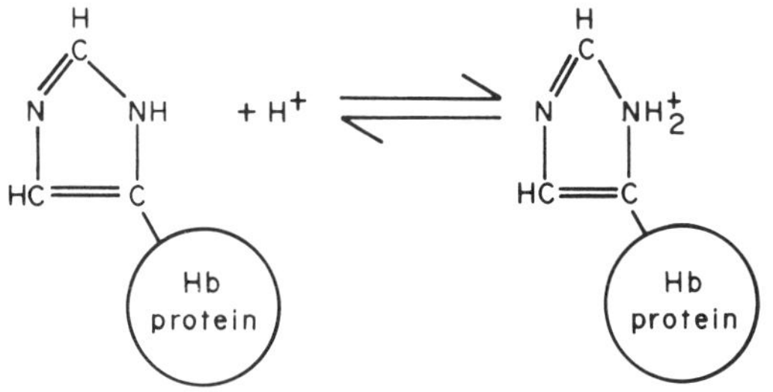

**FIG. 2.** Buffering of $H^+$ by imidazole groups of Hb. (Redrawn from Davenport, H. W.: *The ABC of Acid-Base Chemistry,* 4th Ed., University of Chicago Press, Chicago, 1958.)

of the $HCO_3^-$ ions formed in the red cells, therefore, end up in the plasma. This movement of anions changes the membrane potential somewhat, making the inside less negative relative to the outside, and causes a movement of $Cl^-$ ions from plasma to red cells; this is called the Chloride Shift, or Hamburger Shift. This exchange of $HCO_3^-$ and $Cl^-$ ions is possible within the small amount of time blood spends in the tissues and within the fraction of a second that it spends in the lungs because the red cell membranes are extremely permeable to anions, much more so than most other cell membranes. The extra $HCO_3^-$ and $Cl^-$ ions within the red cells cause water to move from plasma to red cells, and the cells thus swell somewhat. The packed cell volume, or hematocrit, determined in venous blood will therefore be greater than that determined in arterial blood.

While all this $CO_2$ is moving from tissues to blood, $O_2$ is moving from blood to tissues. Figure 1 shows that $HbO_2$ is being deoxygenated to Hb, thus releasing $O_2$ to the tissues at the same time as other parts of the Hb molecule are forming carbamino Hb and binding $H^+$ ions from the $CO_2$ moving from tissues to blood. The Hb molecule is beautifully designed to coordinate these activities. Remember that the binding of $O_2$ and $H^+$ to Hb is a reciprocal one. That is, as $H^+$ binds to Hb, it makes the $O_2$ binding less strong and shifts the curve to the right, resulting in the Bohr shift; as Hb becomes deoxygenated, it binds $H^+$ more strongly and becomes a weaker acid, shifting its pK. Thus, the deoxygenation of Hb which occurs at the tissues, if unaccompanied by any $CO_2$ being taken up (and $H^+$ being released), would cause $H^+$ to be taken up by the Hb and would make the blood more alkaline. This change in pK enables Hb to bind most of the $H^+$ being released as $CO_2$ is taken up by the blood without any change in pH. In fact, for each mole of $O_2$ given off to tissues from Hb, approximately 0.7 mole of $H^+$ can be bound to the Hb without any change in pH. Of course, the respiratory quotient (R.Q.) is normally greater than 0.7, but not much (0.85, or so), so this ability of Hb to change its pK as it becomes deoxygenated is important in minimizing the change in pH of blood as gas exchange occurs at the tissues.

## CO₂ DISSOCIATION CURVE OF BLOOD

One can construct a "CO₂ dissociation curve" using axes similar to those used in the last chapter for the $O_2$ dissociation curve. Both curves are plotted on the same set of axes in Fig. 3; the ordinate is $O_2$ or $CO_2$ content and the abcissa is $Po_2$ or $Pco_2$. The points marked a and $\bar{v}$ on both curves signify the normal arterial and mixed venous blood values, respectively.

## MORE CO₂ CARRIED IN BODY STORES THAN O₂

Viewing the two curves together reveals some major differences between them. First, there is far more $CO_2$ than $O_2$ in every liter of blood. The arterial blood, for instance, whose $Pa_{O_2} = 100$ mm Hg and whose $Pa_{CO_2} = 40$ mm Hg, carries about 200 ml $O_2$/liter and 480 ml $CO_2$/liter. Normal mixed venous blood ($P\bar{v}_{O_2} = 40$ mm Hg, $P\bar{v}_{CO_2} = 48$ mm Hg) carries 150 ml $O_2$/liter and 520 ml

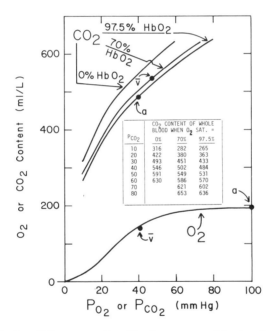

FIG. 3. $CO_2$ and $O_2$ dissociation curves. **Top:** The three curves at the top show the relationship between $CO_2$ content of whole blood and its $Pco_2$; this relationship varies with changes in saturation of Hb with $O_2$. Thus, $Pco_2$ of blood influences $O_2$ saturation (Bohr effect), and $O_2$ saturation of blood influences $CO_2$ content (Haldane effect). The data are tabulated in the *inset.* (Data of Dill, D. B., et al.: *J. Biol. Chem.* 118(3):635, 1937.) **Bottom:** The bottom curve shows the relationship between $O_2$ content on Hb and $Po_2$ from the data tabulated in the previous chapter. Note that the $O_2$ curve has both flat and steep parts in the range between the normal arterial (a) and mixed venous ($\bar{v}$) points, while the $CO_2$ curve is essentially rectilinear in that range. Note also that the $CO_2$ content of blood is far greater than the $O_2$ content in their respective normal ranges, and the $CO_2$ curve is far steeper than that for $O_2$.

$CO_2$/liter. When one considers the whole body stores of these two gases, the difference is even more pronounced.

The major body stores of $O_2$ are in the lungs and blood, with a small amount in muscle myoglobin (a pigment similar to Hb). The total amount stored is about 1.5 liters, which could keep normal resting metabolism going for a maximum of about 6 minutes. $CO_2$ is also carried in the lungs and blood, but by far the major part of the stores is located elsewhere in the body. For instance, the normal person has about 14 liters of extracellular fluid whose $[HCO_3^-]$ is about 25 mEq/liter. Bone, too, carries huge stores of $CO_2$. The total body stores of $CO_2$ have been estimated to be as large as 120 liters when $Pa_{CO_2}$ is about 40 mm Hg and $P\bar{v}_{CO_2}$ is about 48 mm Hg.

Suppose a normal person whose $Pa_{O_2}$ and $Pa_{CO_2}$ begin at nice normal values of 100 and 40 mm Hg, respectively, is asked to double his alveolar ventilation and maintain it there. We know that, in the new steady state, his $Pa_{O_2}$ will be 125 mm Hg and his $Pa_{CO_2}$ will be 20 mm Hg, assuming that his metabolism remains as it was. How long will it take for the new steady state to develop? The $O_2$ stores of the body can approach new steady-state values rather quickly; probably within a minute or so the $PA_{O_2}$ and the $Pa_{O_2}$ would be nearing 125 mm Hg and the various $O_2$ reservoirs would have become filled somewhat more fully as a result of the increased $Po_2$. The $CO_2$ stores of the body would not truly reach a new steady state for weeks! Many liters of $CO_2$ from the stores must be excreted via the lungs before the $CO_2$ stores are in "equilibrium" with the new, lower values of $Pco_2$ throughout the body. Some of these stores, notably bone, exchange rather poorly with blood, and tend to give the process a long, slow tail.

In the process of reaching a new steady state, while $CO_2$ from the body stores is being excreted, the respiratory exchange ratio, R, would be elevated and would not accurately reflect the true R.Q. The R.Q., of course, is equal to the metabolic production of $CO_2$ divided by the metabolic consumption of $O_2$ ($\dot{V}_{CO_2}/\dot{V}_{O_2}$), while R is equal to the amount of $CO_2$ crossing the alveolar membranes per minute divided by the amount of $O_2$ crossing the alveolar membranes per minute. During the approach to the new steady state, the metabolic production of $CO_2$ as well as a considerable amount of $CO_2$ from the body stores would be crossing the alveolar membranes, thus raising the numerator of the equation for R considerably. It is true that the denominator of that equation would be raised also by additional $O_2$ crossing the alveolar membranes to fill the $O_2$ reservoirs somewhat more fully, but the magnitude of this effect is miniscule compared with the $CO_2$. In fact, since the amount of $O_2$ on Hb and myoglobin will not change appreciably, only the lung gas reservoir will fill more fully, and that with less than 0.1 liters of extra $O_2$, while the $CO_2$ reservoirs must empty liters and liters of $CO_2$.

Since R.Q. is determined by measuring R, these considerations have practical importance. One must be sure that one's subject is in a steady state before attempting to determine R.Q., and it is very common for a subject to be hyperventilating somewhat during respiratory procedures to which he is not thoroughly accustomed.

## CO₂ DISSOCIATION CURVE FAIRLY RECTILINEAR IN NORMAL RANGE; O₂ CURVE IS CURVILINEAR

A second significant difference between the two curves is their shape. The $CO_2$ curve is essentially rectilinear in its normal working range of perhaps 30–50 mm Hg; even outside this range, the $CO_2$ content changes with changing $P_{CO_2}$ with roughly a constant slope. The $O_2$ curve is decidedly S-shaped, but has become essentially horizontal at $P_{O_2}$ near the normal alveolar $P_{O_2}$ of 100 mm Hg. This contrast between the two curves is a main ingredient in bringing about situations in which $P_{A_{CO_2}}$ and $P_{a_{CO_2}}$ may not differ grossly from one another, while $P_{A_{O_2}}$ and $P_{a_{O_2}}$ have very different values. An example follows which is depicted schematically in Fig. 4. We assume that the left mainstem

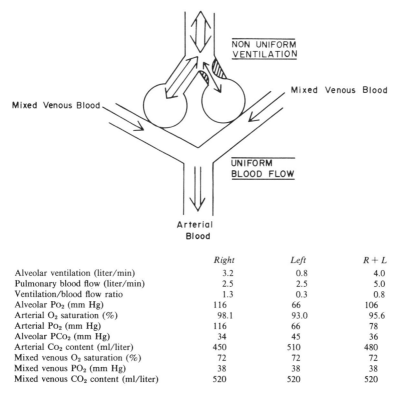

|  | Right | Left | R + L |
|---|---|---|---|
| Alveolar ventilation (liter/min) | 3.2 | 0.8 | 4.0 |
| Pulmonary blood flow (liter/min) | 2.5 | 2.5 | 5.0 |
| Ventilation/blood flow ratio | 1.3 | 0.3 | 0.8 |
| Alveolar Po₂ (mm Hg) | 116 | 66 | 106 |
| Arterial O₂ saturation (%) | 98.1 | 93.0 | 95.6 |
| Arterial Po₂ (mm Hg) | 116 | 66 | 78 |
| Alveolar PCo₂ (mm Hg) | 34 | 45 | 36 |
| Arterial Co₂ content (ml/liter) | 450 | 510 | 480 |
| Mixed venous O₂ saturation (%) | 72 | 72 | 72 |
| Mixed venous PO₂ (mm Hg) | 38 | 38 | 38 |
| Mixed venous CO₂ content (ml/liter) | 520 | 520 | 520 |

**FIG. 4.** A case of uniform blood flow and nonuniform ventilation to the two lungs showing the large difference that can develop between alveolar and arterial Po₂. The difference that develops for Pco₂ is much smaller. The total alveolar ventilation, pulmonary blood flow, and overall V̇ₐ/Q̇ ratio are normal.

bronchus has been partially occluded so that the left lung gets only one-fifth of the alveolar ventilation and the right lung gets four-fifths of the alveolar ventilation, for a total alveolar ventilation that is normal at 4 liters/min. We assume further that the pulmonary blood flow is evenly divided between the two lungs, so that 2.5 liters/min goes to each, again for a total flow that is normal at 5.0 liters/min. The ventilation/blood flow ratios of the two lungs will be abnormal, but the overall ratio is normal at 0.8 (see Chapter 7 for the discussion of ventilation/perfusion ratios). Clearly, $P_{A_{O_2}}$ will be higher—and $P_{A_{CO_2}}$ will be lower—in the right lung than in the left one, and thus the blood perfusing the right lung will come into equilibrium with a higher $P_{A_{O_2}}$—and a lower $P_{A_{CO_2}}$—than the blood perfusing the left lung. This higher than normal $P_{A_{O_2}}$ in the right lung will add negligibly small additional amounts of $O_2$ onto the blood perfusing it, because the Hb-$O_2$ curve is quite horizontal in this range. A $P_{A_{O_2}}$ of 116 mm Hg, which we calculate to exist in the right lung, results in an Hb-$O_2$ saturation of about 98.1% rather than the 97.4% which is achieved at a "normal" $P_{A_{O_2}}$ of 100 mm Hg. The $P_{A_{O_2}}$ of 66 mm Hg, which we calculate to exist in the left lung, however, will result in the Hb being only 93% saturated with $O_2$. When these two streams mix, they will have an Hb-$O_2$ saturation of 95.6% (halfway between 98.1 and 93 because the two blood flows are equal), which corresponds to a $P_{a_{O_2}}$ of 78 mm Hg. We can calculate what the "mixed" $P_{A_{O_2}}$ will be by weighting the contributions from the two lungs appropriately as follows: $P_{A_{O_2}} = [66 + (4 \times 116)]/5 = 106$ mm Hg. Thus, the difference between the $P_{A_{O_2}}$ and the $P_{a_{O_2}}$ is 28 mm Hg.

The values of $P_{A_{CO_2}}$ that can be calculated to exist in the right and left lungs are, respectively, 34 and 45 mm Hg. Because of the almost rectilinear curve of $CO_2$, however, the less than normal $CO_2$ content of the blood from the right lung will partially compensate for the greater than normal $CO_2$ content of the blood from the left lung. The mixed stream of blood, therefore, will have a $CO_2$ content and $P_{a_{CO_2}}$ essentially unchanged from the normal at, respectively, 480 ml/liter and 40 mm Hg. (These $CO_2$ calculations were performed with the tabular data in Fig. 3.) The mixed alveolar $P_{CO_2}$ can be calculated in the same manner as the mixed $P_{A_{O_2}}$, by giving proper weight to the differing alveolar ventilations as follows: $P_{A_{CO_2}} = [45 + (4 \times 34)]/5 = 36.2$ mm Hg. So the difference in partial pressure between the alveolar and arterial $P_{CO_2}$ is 4 mm Hg, much smaller than the 28 mm Hg for $O_2$. I should point out here that this is a much larger $P_{A_{CO_2}} - P_{a_{CO_2}}$ difference than one would expect to see in a normal, healthy person. Because of the relative rectilinearity of the $CO_2$ dissociation curve, together with the steep slope of that curve, and because of physiological mechanisms that tend to match blood flow to ventilation in various parts of the lung, the normal person rarely has a discernible difference between $P_{A_{CO_2}}$ and $P_{a_{CO_2}}$.

Figure 3 demonstrates something else about the $CO_2$ dissociation curve of blood which is worth pointing out. Just as the position of the Hb-$O_2$ dissociation curve changed as a result of $CO_2$ being added to the blood (called the Bohr effect and due mostly to the $H^+$ produced), so does the $CO_2$ dissociation curve change position as the degree of oxygenation of the Hb is changed (called the Haldane effect). Thus, blood can hold more $CO_2$ at any given $P_{CO_2}$ as Hb becomes more deoxygenated, probably because the $H^+$ ions produced during the formation of carbamino compounds and $HCO_3^-$ are more avidly bound by Hb, and thus do not build up to levels that stop the formation of these compounds until higher levels of them have been produced.

## REFERENCES

1. Comroe, J. H., Jr. (1974): *Physiology of Respiration,* 2nd Ed., p. 316. Year Book Medical Publishers, Chicago.
2. Farhi, L. E. (1964): Gas stores of the body. In: *Handbook of Physiology, Sect. 3: Respiration,* edited by W. O. Fenn and H. Rahn, Vol. 1, p. 873. American Physiological Society, Washington, D.C.
3. Roughton, F. J. W. (1964): Transport of oxygen and carbon dioxide. In: *Handbook of Physiology, Sect. 3: Respiration,* edited by W. O. Fenn and H. Rahn, Vol. 1, p. 767.

## PROBLEMS

1. $CO_2$ is carried in the blood mostly

   a. as $HCO_3^-$ in red blood cells
   b. dissolved
   c. as carbamino Hb
   d. as $HCO_3^-$ in the plasma
   e. as carbamino compounds with plasma proteins

2. The reactions that allow erythrocytes to carry $CO_2$ from the tissues to the lungs

   a. require the presence of carbonic anhydrase in the plasma
   b. result in movement of $HCO_3^-$ from plasma to the erythrocyte
   c. result in $H^+$ being removed from Hb molecules
   d. result in movement of $Cl^-$ from erythrocyte to plasma
   e. result in movement of $HCO_3^-$ from erythrocyte to plasma

3. R.Q. of the tissues and R at the lungs are equal to one another:

   a. always, because both are equal to the same thing, $\dot{V}_{CO_2}/\dot{V}_{O_2}$
   b. only during the steady state of rest
   c. only during a basal steady state
   d. during exercise
   e. whenever the subject is in a steady state relative to the transport of $CO_2$ and $O_2$ between lungs and tissues

4. A patient's right mainstem bronchus has become totally occluded. Blood flow through this right lung (occluded airway) is 1.00 liter/min. Blood flow

through the left lung is 5.00 liters/min. The patient's mixed venous $P_{CO_2}$ is 46 mm Hg. His $\dot{V}_{O_2}$ is 250 ml/min. His R.Q. is 0.800. Assume the $CO_2$ dissociation curve of the patient's blood is linear with a slope such that $CO_2$ concentration increases 7.00 ml/liter of blood for each mm Hg increase in $P_{CO_2}$. The $P_{CO_2}$ of the blood in this patient's aorta is closest to

a. 40.0 mm Hg
b. 41.3 mm Hg
c. 42.6 mm Hg
d. 43.7 mm Hg
e. 46.0 mm Hg

## ANSWERS

1. You will remember that $CO_2$ is carried in blood in three forms: dissolved, as carbamino compounds, and as $HCO_3^-$. The relative amounts of these forms are, respectively, roughly 5, 5, and 90%. To decide between (a) and (d), recall that, while most of the $HCO_3^-$ is *formed* in the red cells, most of the $HCO_3^-$ ends up in the plasma. Correct answer is (d).

2. Choice (a) is ruled out because there is no carbonic anhydrase in the plasma. Choices (b), (c), and (d) are backward, leaving choice (e) as the correct one.

3. The R.Q. will be equal to the R only when body stores of both $O_2$ and $CO_2$ are remaining constant (when they are being neither filled or emptied). Under these conditions, one molecule of $O_2$ will pass across the alveolar membranes for each molecule of $O_2$ that is used to oxidize foodstuffs in the mitochondria, and one molecule of $CO_2$ will cross the alveolar membranes for each molecule of $CO_2$ that is produced by that process of oxidation. This defines the existence of a steady state for $CO_2$ and $O_2$ transport in which the R.Q. will be equal to the R. Thus, (a) and (d) fail to specify whether a steady state exists, (b) and (c) are too restrictive, and (e) is the correct answer.

4. As shown in Fig. 5, the right mainstem bronchus is occluded, no gas exchange occurs in the right lung. Therefore, the entire $\dot{V}_{CO_2}$ of 200 ml/min (0.8 × 250 ml/min) must exchange in the left lung. The left lung $\dot{Q}$ of 5 liters/min means that 40 ml $CO_2$ must come from each liter. The $CO_2$ dissociation curve slope of (7 ml $CO_2$/liter)/mm Hg means that the pulmonary venous blood coming from the left lung will have a $P_{CO_2}$ of 40.3 mm Hg (5.71 mm Hg lower than the mixed venous $P_{CO_2}$). When 5 liters/min of this blood mix with 1 liter of low from the right lung, the mixed pulmonary venous $P_{CO_2}$ will be 41.3 mm Hg. One can also consider both lungs together.

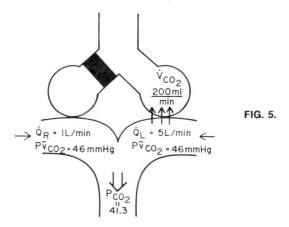

**FIG. 5.**

The total flow is 6 liters/min, which means that the $\dot{V}CO_2$ of 200 ml/min will result in a decreased $CO_2$ content in mixed pulmonary venous blood of $200/6 = 33.33 \ldots$ ml $CO_2$/liter of blood. But the slope of the $CO_2$ dissociation curve is given to be (7 ml $CO_2$/liter of blood)/mm Hg. Thus the mixed pulmonary venous blood $PCO_2$ is lower than the mixed venous $PCO_2$ by $33.33 \ldots /7 = 4.76$ mm Hg. $46 - 4.76 = 41.2$ mm Hg. Either method leads to answer (b).

# 6

---

# *Acid–Base Balance: Disturbances*

A normal person's arterial pH ($pH_a$) is about 7.40, and this $pH_a$ must be kept very constant if normal enzyme function is to be maintained throughout the human body. Surprisingly small deviations from this pH lead to weakness and general physiological disability, and further deviations lead to collapse, coma, and death. In fact, the $pH_a$ range consistent with human life is only about 6.8–7.8, and the normal, healthy, sea-level person's $pH_a$ probably never differs from 7.4 by more than 0.15 pH units.

Much of the explanation for why the $pH_a$ range consistent with life seems so small derives from the units with which we express it: $pH = - \log [H^+]$ (physicians and other scientists frequently use logarithms to make large ranges of variables seem smaller.). A $pH_a$ of 7.40 represents a $[H^+]_a$ of $40 \times 10^{-9}$ Eq/liter, or 40 nEq/liter. The range of $pH_a$ consistent with life would represent $[H^+]_a$ of 158–15.8 nEq/liter, or a 10-fold variation of $[H^+]_a$. There are few important substances whose arterial blood concentration could change by a factor of 10 without being life-threatening.

This chapter begins with a consideration of how one assesses the acid–base status of biological fluids through the use of the $CO_2/HCO_3^-$ buffer system. Next, the characteristics of solutions that contain no buffers other than the $CO_2/HCO_3^-$ system (e.g., CSF) are contrasted with the characteristics of those that have other buffer systems as well (e.g., blood). The Siggaard-Andersen Curve Nomogram is then introduced and used to compare these two types of fluid graphically. The four "pure" acid–base disturbances are then defined and discussed qualitatively. Finally, the Siggaard-Andersen Curve Nomogram is used to quantitate these acid–base disturbances, and to discuss some mixed acid–base disturbances.

## ASSESSMENT OF ACID–BASE STATUS: HENDERSON-HASSELBALCH EQUATION

The Henderson-Hasselbalch equation relates the pH of a solution with the $pK_a$ of a given buffer system and the concentrations of its ionized and unionized forms at equilibrium: $pH = pK_a + \log [A^-]/[HA]$. Thus, for any given buffer system, the ratio of $[A^-]/[HA]$ defines a unique pH. Further, in a solution with many buffers, the various $[A^-]/[HA]$ ratios must all be consistent with the solution's pH. Therefore, it is possible to assess the acid–base status of a fluid sample by determining $[A^-]$ and $[HA]$ for any buffer system, and using that knowledge together with the $pK_a$ of that buffer system. This was the procedure employed before the modern pH electrode came into common use, and it is still a method of choice in assessing acid–base status in fluids not easily reached by a pH electrode (e.g., intracellular fluid). Now that the pH electrode is commonly available and quite dependable, one can simply measure pH, and one of the other two variables ($[A^-]$ or $[HA]$), and calculate the remaining one.

The buffer system that is almost invariably utilized when assessing the acid–base status of human blood is the $CO_2/HCO_3^-$ system. This is so for at least three reasons: (a) Its components are in reasonably high concentration and are easy to analyze. (b) Metabolism pours a steady stream of $CO_2$ into the body, and acid–base disturbance of considerable magnitude is therefore unavoidable if the mechanisms involved in the removal of that $CO_2$ malfunction. (c) Perhaps most important is the fact that the acid–base balance of the body is maintained through the control of the two components of this system: The lungs control $P_{CO_2}$ through the control of alveolar ventilation, and the kidneys control $[HCO_3^-]$. Thus, the Henderson-Hasselbalch equation for this system might be functionally written, pH = pK + log [kidneys]/[lungs], to emphasize this very important third reason.

A somewhat more quantitatively useful form of the Henderson-Hasselbalch equation for this system is

$$pH = pK' + \log \frac{[HCO_3^-]}{[(0.03 \text{ mM/liter})/mm \text{ Hg}]P_{CO_2}}$$

where the numerator of the equation has the units of mEq/liter in plasma and the denominator has the units of mM/liter, and is a concentration of $CO_2$ again in plasma.

Several aspects of this commonly used form of the Henderson-Hasselbalch equation for the $CO_2/HCO_3^-$ system puzzle students, and rightly so. They are, (a) "Why is the denominator a concentration of $CO_2$ in the first place? Shouldn't the fraction read log $[HCO_3^-]/[H_2CO_3]$? (b) "What does pK' mean and why is its value 6.1?" and (c) (for those students with long memories) "Why is the solubility constant for $CO_2$ 0.03, instead of the 0.7 that we used in the previous chapter?" Let me deal with these potentially confusing issues one by one.

Firstly, $[H_2CO_3]$ is not the quantity used in the denominator because it exists in quantities that are too small to be analyzed in normal plasma. The pK of the system is about $3.4 \times 10^{-4}$, so at normal pH of 7.4 there would be only about 0.0024 mEq/liter of $H_2CO_3$. We know, however, that there is a quantitative relationship between $CO_2$ and $H_2CO_3$ at equilibrium. $CO_2 + H_2O \rightleftarrows H_2CO_3$, and $K_{hydration} = [CO_2][H_2O]/[H_2CO_3]$, or $[H_2CO_3] = [CO_2][H_2O]/K_{hydration}$.

Now, since the concentration of $H_2O$ and the $K_{hydration}$ are constants, we can replace the term $[H_2CO_3]$ in the Hendersen-Hasselbalch equation with $[CO_2] \times$ constant.

This leads directly to the second question. As mentioned just above, the actual $K_{dissoc.}$ of the $CO_2/HCO_3^-$ system is about $3.4 \times 10^{-4}$, resulting in an actual pK of about 3.47. The pK' of 6.1, which amounts to a K' of about $8 \times 10^{-7}$, is the result of incorporating the constant that we divided $[CO_2]$ by to get $[H_2CO_3]$ into the dissociation constant; thus, $[CO_2]/418 = [H_2CO_3]$, and $(10^{-3.47})/418 = 10^{-6.09}$. By taking its negative logarithm this K' then becomes 6.09, which is the apparent pK or the pK' of this system.

Thirdly, the solubility constant being used in the Henderson-Hasselbalch equation is 0.03 (mM/liter)/mm Hg. The solubility constant used for $CO_2$ in the previous chapter is 0.7 (ml/liter)/mm Hg, having totally different units. If one multiplies the Henderson-Hasselbalch constant [0.03 (mM/liter)/mm Hg] by the number of ml/mM (22.3), one gets the solubility constant 0.67 (ml/liter)/mm Hg, or about 0.7 (ml/liter)/mm Hg, which was the number and units used in the last chapter.

In normal arterial blood plasma, $P_{CO_2} = 40$ mm Hg and $[HCO_3^-]$ is about 24 mEq/liter. Plugging these values into the Henderson-Hasselbalch equation, we get

$$pH_a = 6.1 + \log \frac{24 \text{ mEq/liter}}{[(0.03 \text{ mM/liter})/\text{mm Hg}](40 \text{ mm Hg})} =$$

$$6.1 + \log \frac{24 \text{ mEq/liter}}{1.2 \text{ mM/liter}} = 6.1 + \log 20/1, pH_a = 6.1 + 1.3 = 7.4$$

Note that the pH of this plasma or any other solution will be 7.4 whenever the ratio of $[HCO_3^-]/[CO_2]$ is 20/1, regardless of what the individual values of the numerator and denominator are. This provides a quick and easy way to assess whether the pH of a sample is that of normal, sea-level arterial blood (7.4, ratio 20/1), or whether it is more acid than that (< 7.4, ratio < 20/1), or whether it is more alkaline than that (> 7.4, ratio > 20/1). If an arterial blood sample is more acid than 7.4, the condition is called acidemia, or acidosis; an arterial sample that is more alkaline than 7.4 means that the donor is alkalemic, or alkalotic.

## SOLUTIONS IN WHICH THE $CO_2/HCO_3^-$ BUFFER SYSTEM IS THE ONLY IMPORTANT ONE (e.g., CSF)

Let us now follow the acid–base status of a solution such as CSF in which the $CO_2/HCO_3^-$ buffer system is the only important one, as we change the $P_{CO_2}$ with which that solution is in equilibrium. If we raise $P_{CO_2}$, for instance, we will cause $CO_2$ to hydrate to form $H_2CO_3$, which will then dissociate into $H^+$ and $HCO_3^-$ as follows: $CO_2 + H_2O \rightleftarrows H_2CO_3 \rightleftarrows H^+ + HCO_3^-$. In fact, in

TABLE 1. *Effects of adding CO₂ to fluids with and without buffers other than bicarbonate*

| Type of Fluid | [HCO₃⁻] (mEq/liter) | pH | [H⁺] (nEq/liter) | Pco₂ (mm Hg) | |
|---|---|---|---|---|---|
| **A.** Fluid with no nonbicarbonate | 24.2 | 7.6 | 25 | 25 | INITIAL |
| buffers of importance (CSF) | 24.2 | 7.2 | 63 | 63 | FINAL |
| **B.** Fluid with buffers in addition | 20 | 7.55 | 28 | 23 | INITIAL |
| to bicarbonate (blood) | 30 | 7.25 | 56 | 70 | FINAL |

such a solution, every molecule of $CO_2$ that hydrates and dissociates will form one $H^+$ and one $HCO_3^-$ ion; in such a solution, therefore, the change in $[H^+]$ and the change in $[HCO_3^-]$ must be exactly equal.

Table 1A shows the acid–base data that might result from this type of solution as $P_{CO_2}$ is increased. It shows data before $P_{CO_2}$ is raised (INITIAL) and after it is raised (FINAL). It seems surprising at first glance that $[HCO_3^-]$ has not changed even though $P_{CO_2}$ has been increased by a factor of 2.5, making the solution considerably more acid ($[H^+]$ increased by factor of 2.5, pH goes from 7.6 to 7.2). Isn't it true that, as a result of the addition of $CO_2$, one $HCO_3^-$ ion is produced in this type of solution for every $H^+$ ion produced? The answer is yes, of course, and the reason that $[HCO_3^-]$ does not seem to change (although it does, slightly) is that its concentration is almost a million times greater than the $H^+$ concentration at the outset. Remember that $[HCO_3^-]$ initially is $24.2 \times 10^{-3}$ Eq/liter whereas $[H^+]$ initially is $25 \times 10^{-9}$ Eq/liter.

One can use the "nonlog form" of the Henderson-Hasselbalch equation to quantitate this acid–base transition (actually, of course, the Henderson-Hasselbalch equation is derived from this nonlog statement of the dissociation equilibrium). $K' = [HCO_3^-][H^+]/0.03 (P_{CO_2})$. The INITIAL values look like this:

$$10^{-6.1} = \frac{24.2 \times 10^{-3} \text{ Eq/liter} (25 \times 10^{-9} \text{ Eq/liter})}{[(0.03 \times 10^{-3} \text{ M/liter})/\text{mm Hg}] (25 \text{ mm Hg})}$$

and

$$10^{-6.1} = 10^{-6.1}.$$

Let us now look at the same relationship after we raise the $P_{CO_2}$ to 63 mm Hg. That will raise the denominator by a factor of 2.5; clearly the numerator must also go up by a factor of 2.5 before the system will once again be in equilibrium. That equilibrium occurs when $38 \times 10^{-9}$ M/liter of $CO_2$ have "moved to the right" through $H_2CO_3$ to $HCO_3^-$ and $H^+$, giving the FINAL values shown in Table 1A. Plugging these values into the statement of the dissociation equilibrium gives:

$$10^{-6.1} = \frac{24.200038 \times 10^{-3} \text{ Eq/liter} (63 \times 10^{-9} \text{ Eq/liter})}{[(0.03 \times 10^{-3} \text{ M/liter})/\text{mm Hg}] (63 \text{ mm Hg})}$$

and,

$$10^{-6.1} = 10^{-6.1}.$$

The numerator has increased by a factor of 2.5 by virture of $[H^+]$ having increased by a factor of 2.5, before $[HCO_3^-]$ has changed at all measurably. The bottom line reads as follows: Solutions whose only buffer system is the $CO_2/HCO_3^-$ system are isobicarbonate solutions as $CO_2$ is added or taken away. (This statement is true for all solutions of biological import. You could, however, add $CO_2$ to distilled water, producing large *percentage* changes in $[HCO_3^-]$, although the absolute amount of the changes would still be immeasurably small.)

It is worth noting that large changes in pH were induced in this type of solution as $P_{CO_2}$ was changed. The $CO_2/HCO_3^-$ system is not effective in buffering against changes in pH that are induced through the addition of $CO_2$. The reader is urged to compare the behavior of this type of solution with that of a solution such as blood, which contains other, potent buffer systems (to be discussed next).

## SOLUTIONS THAT CONTAIN BUFFERS IN ADDITION TO THE $CO_2/HCO_3^-$ SYSTEM (BLOOD)

As mentioned in the last chapter, the plasma proteins and especially the hemoglobin of blood are potent buffers. In addition to these, and to the $CO_2/HCO_3^-$ system, blood also has small amounts of $HPO_4^{2-}/H_2PO_4^-$ and many other lesser buffer systems. If we added $CO_2$ to a fluid such as this, $CO_2$ would hydrate to form $H_2CO_3$, which in turn would dissociate to form $H^+$ and $HCO_3^-$ ions as in the previous solution. But, there is a difference! The $H^+$ ions, rather than remaining free in solution, are mostly bound to protein buffers (Pr), as follows:

$$CO_2 + H_2O \rightleftarrows H_2CO_3 \rightleftarrows HCO_3^- + H^+$$
$$+$$
$$Pr^-$$
$$\upharpoonleft\downharpoonright$$
$$HPr$$

(Table 1B shows the data that one might get from a solution of normal human blood as its $P_{CO_2}$ was raised from 23 to 70 mm Hg, a three-fold increase.) Let us again write the nonlog dissociation equilibrium equation in the INITIAL STATE:

$$K' = \frac{[HCO_3^-][H^+]}{0.03\ (P_{CO_2})}$$

$$10^{-6.1} = \frac{20 \times 10^{-3}\ \text{Eq/liter}\ (28 \times 10^{-9}\ \text{Eq/liter})}{[(0.03 \times 10^{-3}\ \text{M/liter})/\text{mm Hg}]\ (23\ \text{mm Hg})}$$

or, again, $10^{-6.1} = 10^{-6.1}$. Between the initial and final states, we have increased $P_{CO_2}$ and therefore $[CO_2]$ by a factor of three. If the denominator increases by a factor of three, the numerator must increase by a factor of three to satisfy the same $K'$. Enough $CO_2$ molecules must hydrate and subsequently dissociate to raise the product $[HCO_3^-][H^+]$ by a factor of three. In this solution, however, most of the $H^+$ ions are "scrubbed up" by the proteins, so that many, many more $CO_2$ molecules can move through the hydration and dissociation to form many, many more $H^+$ and $HCO_3^-$ ions than were formed in the previous solution. So many $HCO_3^-$ ions are formed that $[HCO_3^-]$ changes markedly from 20 mEq/liter INITIALLY to 30 mEq/liter FINALLY. In the FINAL state, the dissociation equilibrium equation looks thus:

$$10^{-6.1} = \frac{30 \times 10^{-3} \text{ Eq/liter } (56 \times 10^{-9} \text{ Eq/liter})}{[(0.03 \times 10^{-3} \text{ M/liter})/\text{mm Hg}] (70 \text{ mm Hg})}$$

or

$$10^{-6.1} = 10^{-6.1}.$$

Both denominator and numerator have increased by a factor of three; the numerator's increase in this case consists of a 1.5-fold increase in $[HCO_3^-]$ (from 20 to 30 mEq/liter) and a 2-fold increase in $[H^+]$, (from 28 to 56 nEq/liter). A "take-home" message here is that when one changes the $P_{CO_2}$ of a solution like blood, which has effective buffers in addition to $CO_2/HCO_3^-$, $[HCO_3^-]$ also changes.

A related and equally important conclusion to be drawn from the comparison of these two solutions is that a fluid like blood is far better protected against changes in pH when $CO_2$ is added or removed than is a fluid such as CSF. The $P_{CO_2}$ of the CSF was increased by a factor of 2.5 which led to a fall in pH of 0.4 units. The $P_{CO_2}$ of the blood was increased by a factor of 3, leading to a fall in pH of only 0.3 units. The reason for this better protection is, of course, that the protein buffers of blood are very effective in "scrubbing up" $H^+$ ions released by the addition of $CO_2$. We can see just how effective they are by comparing the large total number of $H^+$ ions formed by this threefold increase in $P_{CO_2}$ with the small increase in free $H^+$ ions which results. Since each $CO_2$ molecule that moves "to the right" through hydration and dissociation forms both an $HCO_3^-$ ion and an $H^+$ ion, the total numbers of each formed must be equal. Since $[HCO_3^-]$ increased by 10 mEq/liter, 10 mEq of $H^+$ ions also must have released into each liter of blood. Concentration of $H^+$ ions increased from 28 to 56 nEq/liter, a change of 28 nEq/liter. So the ratio of total $H^+$ ions formed to increase in free $H^+$ ions is $(10 \times 10^{-3} \text{ Eq/liter})/(28 \times 10^{-9} \text{ Eq/liter})$, or about 1,000,000/3. That is, for every million $H^+$ ions produced as $CO_2$ is added to blood, 999,997 are bound to blood proteins, and only 3 are allowed to remain free in solution!

## THE SIGGAARD-ANDERSEN CURVE NOMOGRAM

Several different types of graphs have been used to plot the three variables of the Henderson-Hasselbalch equation: pH, $P_{CO_2}$, and $[HCO_3^-]$. Generally, one of these variables is plotted against one of the others, and the third variable becomes a series of lines across the graph. Each of these lines defines all the points of a given $[HCO_3^-]$, or a given $P_{CO_2}$, or a given pH. The Siggaard-Andersen curve Nomogram is perhaps the most commonly used today, and a modified version of that nomogram is shown in Fig. 1. The log of $P_{CO_2}$ forms the ordinate and the pH (which is the negative log of $[H^+]$) forms the abscissa, and the $[HCO_3^-]$ is displayed as a series of straight lines whose slopes are $-45°$ if one log unit is represented by the same distance on ordinate and abscissa.

The data from Table 1 have been plotted on this nomogram. The INITIAL and FINAL points of solution A, the CSF, have been plotted as points $A_I$ and $A_F$. As the $P_{CO_2}$ of the CSF was raised from 25 to 63, causing a fall in pH from 7.6 to 7.2, a "$CO_2$ titration line" is traced on the graph just slightly below the line of $[HCO_3^-] = 25$ mEq/liter (actually, the value is 24.2 mEq/liter) and parallel to it. $[HCO_3^-]$ did not change in this fluid as $P_{CO_2}$ was raised, so the $CO_2$ titration line has a slope of $-45°$; it is an isobicarbonate line at $[HCO_3^-] = 24.2$ mEq/liter.

The INITIAL and FINAL points of solution B, the blood, have been plotted as $B_I$ and $B_F$. $P_{CO_2}$ was raised from 23 to 70 mm Hg, causing a fall in pH from 7.55 to 7.25, and tracing out a $CO_2$ titration line which is much steeper than that of solution A. The increased steepness of the blood's $CO_2$ titration line means that blood is better protected against changes in pH as its $P_{CO_2}$ is changed than is CSF. A given change in $P_{CO_2}$ produces a smaller change in pH in blood than it does in CSF. The steep slope also means that $[HCO_3^-]$ in this fluid changes as its $P_{CO_2}$ is changed; its $CO_2$ titration line crosses isobicarbonate lines. Point $B_I$ is on the line whose $[HCO_3^-] = 20$, and point $B_F$ is on the line whose $[HCO_3^-] = 30$.

## THE FOUR "PURE" ACID–BASE DISORDERS

The acid–base status of normal arterial blood can be altered in two general ways: (a) By raising or lowering $P_{A_{CO_2}}$, which results in a Respiratory Acidosis or Alkalosis, respectively, and (b) by adding or removing acids other than $H_2CO_3$, which will produce, respectively, a Metabolic Acidosis or Alkalosis. Let us briefly consider the primary events initiating each of these disturbances, and the changes in $[H^+]$, $[HCO_3^-]$, and $P_{A_{CO_2}}$ that might result.

Table 2 shows the series of reactions involved in the hydration of $CO_2$ and the subsequent dissociation of $H_2CO_3$ together with the changes (from normal) in the concentrations of $CO_2$, $HCO_3^-$, and $H^+$ which exist during each of the four "pure" acid–base disturbances. (Although "pure" acid–base disturbances

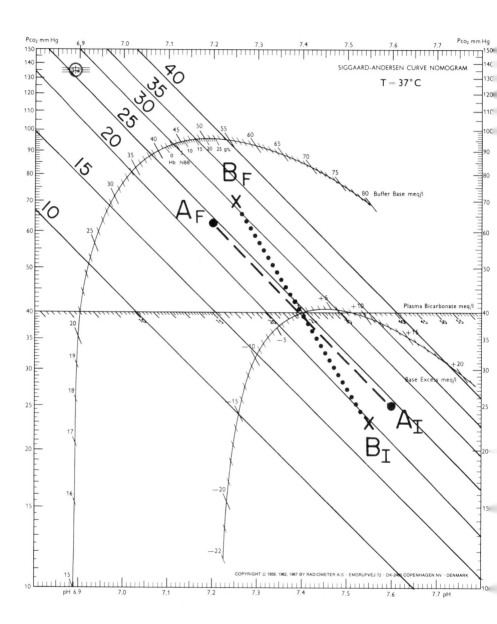

TABLE 2. *Changes in $CO_2$ concentration, $[HCO_3^-]$, and $[H^+]$ occurring during various acid–base disturbances[a]*

| | $H_2O + CO_2 \rightleftarrows H_2CO_3 \rightleftarrows HCO_3^- + H^+$ | | |
|---|---|---|---|
| Respiratory acidosis | ↑* | ↑ | ↑ |
| Respiratory alkalosis | ↓* | ↓ | ↓ |
| Metabolic acidosis | ↓ | ↓* | ↑* |
| Metabolic alkalosis | ± ↑ | ↑* | ↓* |

[a] The primary or initiating event(s) are asterisked in each case.

are rare, their consideration helps the beginning student.) In addition, an asterisk is placed next to the change in concentration which is the initiating event in each pure disturbance.

### Respiratory Acidosis—Pure

The primary or initiating event in respiratory acidosis is an increase in the $CO_2$ concentration, which must itself have been caused by an increase in the $P_{CO_2}$. You will remember that $P_{CO_2}$ increases when the ratio $\dot{V}_{CO_2}/\dot{V}_A$ increases above the normal of about 1/21.5. So, anything that increases $\dot{V}_{CO_2}$ without a corresponding increase in $\dot{V}_A$, or that decreases $\dot{V}_A$ without $\dot{V}_{CO_2}$ having decreased, will inevitably raise $P_{A_{CO_2}}$, $P_{a_{CO_2}}$, and $P_{CO_2}$ throughout the body, thus raising $[CO_2]$ in plasma and elsewhere. As we already know, increasing $[CO_2]$ causes $CO_2$ molecules to "move to the right" through hydration and dissociation, forming more $HCO_3^-$ and $H^+$. A "pure" respiratory acidosis, therefore, will have concentrations of $CO_2$, $HCO_3^-$, and $H^+$ that are higher than "normal."

### Respiratory Alkalosis—Pure

The initiating event in respiratory alkalosis is a decrease in $P_{CO_2}$, caused by a decrease of the ratio $\dot{V}_{CO_2}/\dot{V}_A$ below the normal of about 1/21.5. This causes $HCO_3^-$ and $H^+$ to associate and move to the left through the series of reactions. Thus, in a pure respiratory alkalosis, the concentrations of $CO_2$, $HCO_3^-$ and $H^+$ will be lower than normal.

FIG. 1. A modified Siggaard-Andersen Curve Nomogram comparing the $CO_2$ titration curve of a fluid whose only buffer system is the $CO_2/HCO_3^-$ system ($A_I–A_F$) with that of a fluid containing significant protein buffers in addition ($B_I–B_F$). The curve of the former fluid is less steep than that of the latter; in other words, for any given change in $P_{CO_2}$, the pH of the former fluid changes more than that of the latter. Fluid B (which is normal blood) is better buffered against changes in pH caused by changes in $P_{CO_2}$ than is fluid A (whose buffering characteristics are approached by normal CSF). (Reproduced with permission from *Radiometer*, Copenhagen.)

### Metabolic Acidosis

A primary event causing metabolic acidosis is an increase in $[H^+]$ brought about by the addition of an acid other than $H_2CO_3$ to body fluids (HCl, lactic acid, acetoacetic acid, $\beta$-OH butyric acid, etc.). Many of these $H^+$ ions will associate with $HCO_3^-$ ions, move to the left through the series of reactions, and be quickly lost as $CO_2$ via the lungs. The increased acidity will tend to increase ventilation (through mechanisms that will be discussed in subsequent chapters), and as a result, the $Pco_2$ will be lower than "normal." Thus, this initiating event will result in decreased concentrations of $CO_2$ and $HCO_3^-$, and an increased $H^+$ concentration.

Another initiating event tending to produce metabolic acidosis is the loss of $HCO_3^-$ ions from the body. Prolonged diarrhea may be the means by which this occurs. Again looking at Table 2, we can see that a primary decrease in $[HCO_3^-]$ will pull $CO_2$ through the series of reactions to the right, forming $H^+$ ions, and therefore making body fluids acid. The acidity will again stimulate ventilation, lowering $Pco_2$. Thus again, the concentrations of $CO_2$ and $HCO_3^-$ will be low, and the $H^+$ concentration high.

It should be pointed out that a metabolic acidosis is almost never "pure," since the acidity stimulates ventilation which lowers $Pco_2$. Only in the case of a patient whose ventilatory response to acidity is abolished might one see the "pure" case. This abolition could occur if the sensors normally responsive to $H^+$ were inoperative, if the CNS were unresponsive to the input of these receptors, or if the respiratory muscles themselves were paralyzed, the patient being ventilated mechanically.

### Metabolic Alkalosis

The initiating events which cause metabolic alkalosis are the opposites of those causing metabolic acidosis; either the loss of an acid other than $H_2CO_3$ from the body (a concentrated solution of HCl can be lost via prolonged vomiting) or the addition of $HCO_3^-$ ions to the body fluids (an excessive intake of antacid tablets, perhaps). As in metabolic acidosis, either initial event causes the other to occur. If $H^+$ ions are lost, then $CO_2$ moves to the right through the series of reactions, raising $[HCO_3^-]$; if $HCO_3^-$ ions are added, then some $H^+$ react with the $HCO_3^-$, lowering the $[H^+]$. In either case, the alkalosis tends to decrease ventilation, raising $Pco_2$, but the effect is not a large one. That is, changes in acidity on the alkaline side of "normal" tend to have less effect on ventilation than do changes in acidity on the acid side of "normal." Thus, $Pco_2$ may go up somewhat, or it may not change much. The end result is that the concentrations of $CO_2$ and $HCO_3^-$ are elevated, and the $H^+$ concentration is lowered.

## ACID–BASE STATES ON SIGGAARD—ANDERSEN CURVE NOMOGRAM

Let us return to Fig. 1. You will recall that line $B_I$–$B_F$ traces the path of normal arterial blood as its $P_{CO_2}$ is changed from 23 to 70 mm Hg. That line passes through the point representing the normal values for arterial blood (pH = 7.4, $P_{CO_2}$ = 40 mm Hg, $[HCO_3^-]$ = 24.2 mEq/liter). The acid–base values of any sample of normal blood having a "pure" respiratory acidosis or alkalosis must lie on this line (or on extensions of it). Thus, point $B_F$ represents a sample of blood with pure respiratory acidosis and point $B_I$ represents a sample of blood with pure respiratory alkalosis.

The acid–base values of a sample of "normal" blood having metabolic acidosis or alkalosis must lie off this line; metabolic acidosis to its left and metabolic alkalosis to its right. Pure metabolic acid–base disturbances must lie on the $P_{CO_2}$ = 40 mm Hg line, since only those samples will have no respiratory acid–base disturbance. So, pure metabolic acidosis is on that line to the left of pH = 7.4, and pure metabolic alkalosis is on the line to the right of pH = 7.4.

### Metabolic Acidosis With Respiratory Compensation

Of course, we have already shown that "pure" metabolic acidoses and alkaloses cannot exist in persons whose respiratory responses to $H^+$ concentration are normal; ventilation quickly changes, adding a component of respiratory compensation. It is called respiratory *compensation* because the change in ventilation and subsequent change in $P_{CO_2}$ moves the pH back toward normal. This sequence can be seen in Fig. 2, which is another Siggaard-Andersen Curve Nomogram, this time without the lines of isobicarbonate concentration. The point designated $N$ is at the normal, sea-level, acid–base status of arterial blood, pH = 7.4, $P_{CO_2}$ = 40 mm Hg. Through this point is drawn the nornal blood buffer line (NBBL), which includes all the acid–base values of normal blood having a pure respiratory acidosis (up to the left) or alkalosis (down to the right). You will notice that two curves are included in the nomogram that were left out of Fig. 1, a Buffer Base-Hb concentration curve and a Base Excess curve. The slope of this normal buffer line was defined by drawing the line through the normal point $N$ and through the Hb concentration = 15 g% = 15 g/100 ml = 150 g/liter. This should make sense if the reader remembers that the amount of Hb in blood determines how well buffered that blood is against $CO_2$-induced changes in pH. Thus, higher [Hb] means steeper blood buffer line, and vice versa.

Let us begin with normal arterial blood acid–base status at the point $N$ and induce a pure metabolic acidosis by adding HCl to an anesthetized animal whose ventilation is being kept constant. This will take us to the point $M^1$

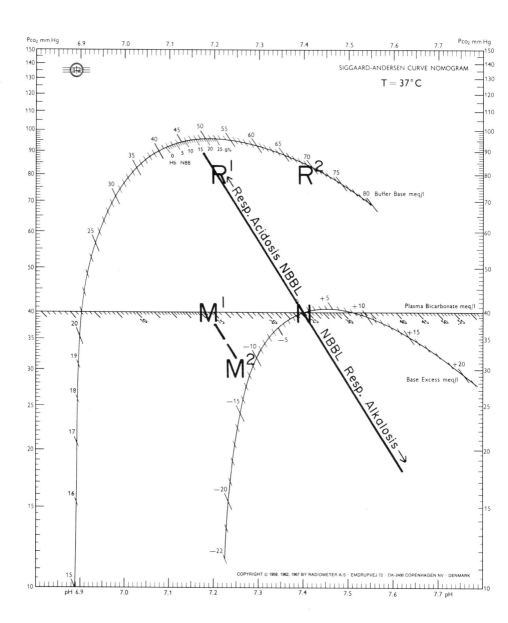

whose pH = 7.2 at a $P_{CO_2}$ which is still 40 mm Hg. If we now allow ventilation to change in response to the considerable acidity of blood and body fluids, the values move to point $M^2$. The ventilation has increased by perhaps four-thirds, lowering $P_{CO_2}$ to about three-fourths of what it was, or to 30 mm Hg. This has resulted in the blood pH rising to 7.25, moving partway back toward "normal" of 7.4, and effecting a respiratory compensation to a metabolic acidosis.

It should be pointed out clearly that the respiratory compensation to a metabolic acid–base disturbance cannot restore the disturbance to normal. Only the kidney can do that. In fact, the respiratory compensation, in the process of partially restoring the pH toward normal, pushed $[HCO_3^-]$ even farther from normal. Point $N$ has a $[HCO_3^-]$ of about 24.2 mEq/liter, and point $M^1$ has had its $[HCO_3^-]$ lowered to 15 mEq/liter. The respiratory compensation, moving from $M^1$ to $M^2$, cuts across isobicarbonate lines, so that point $M^1$ has a $[HCO_3^-]$ of about 12.5 mEq/liter.

### Respiratory Acidosis With Renal Compensation

Although any point representing an acute respiratory acidosis must lie on the blood buffer line above the line of $P_{CO_2}$ = 40 mm Hg, the blood acid–base status will change with time even though $P_{CO_2}$ may be maintained constant. The renal compensation to a respiratory acid–base disturbance again pushes $[HCO_3^-]$ even farther from normal in the process of returning the pH toward normal. Let us return to Fig. 2 and induce a respiratory acidosis represented by point $R^1$. The pH of this point is 7.22, its $P_{CO_2}$ is 80 mm Hg, and its $[HCO_3^-]$ is almost 32 mEq/liter. If we maintain this $P_{CO_2}$ for days or weeks, adding sufficient $O_2$ to the inspired gas to prevent hypoxia, the kidneys will generate new $HCO_3^-$ and thus raise the blood $[HCO_3^-]$ until the ratio of $[HCO_3^-]/[CO_2]$ is 20/1, as it was in the normal state represented by point $N$. If this ratio is 20/1, then the blood pH must be normal at 7.4. Since $[CO_2]$ is two times normal, $[HCO_3^-]$ must also be two times normal, and must be equal to about 48 mEq/liter. When this renal compensation is complete (point $R^2$), the pH may well be normal, although $P_{CO_2}$ and $[HCO_3^-]$ are decidedly not. Just as it was impossible for respiratory compensation to completely restore a metabolic acid–base disturbance to normal, the kidneys cannot restore a respiratory acid–base disturbance completely to normal. A respiratory disturbance

---

**FIG. 2.** Respiratory acidosis and its renal compensation; metabolic acidosis and its respiratory compensation. Point *N* is the normal point on the normal blood buffer line (NBBL). Pure respiratory acidosis is represented by moving up the NBBL to point $R^1$; with the time, renal compensation adds $HCO_3^-$, eventuating in point $R^2$. Again from point *N*, the development of a pure metabolic acidosis is represented by movement to point $M^1$; allowing respiration to respond to that acidosis causes respiratory compensation, moving to point $M^2$. Note that the renal compensation to a respiratory acidosis can return blood pH essentially to normal. The respiratory compensation to a metabolic acidosis can never do so, returning the pH only part-way back toward normal. (Reproduced with permission from *Radiometer*, Copenhagen.)

can only be restored completely to normal by adjusting pulmonary function in such a way as to restore $P_{CO_2}$ to normal.

Note that the renal compensation to respiratory acid–base disturbances differs from the respiratory compensation to metabolic acid–base disturbances in two major ways: (a) It is far slower, taking days or weeks to reach completion, and (b) it can and does restore the pH completely to normal, whereas the respiratory compensation only restores the pH part way back toward normal. The two types of compensation are similar in that they shift $[HCO_3^-]$ even farther from normal in the process of restoring the pH back toward normal.

### Acute Emergencies Involving Both Respiratory and Metabolic Acidosis

A serious acid–base disturbance as well as extreme tissue hypoxia can quickly develop in respiratory arrest. Tissue metabolism continues to pour $CO_2$ into tissues and lung gases, but there is no alveolar ventilation to wash the $CO_2$ into the environment (thus, respiratory acidosis). Tissue metabolism also continues to utilize $O_2$ from very limited stores (remember that, at the end of a normal breath, there is only enough $O_2$ in body stores to support normal resting metabolism for 4–6 minutes, even assuming that all of the stores could be used). The decreasing $O_2$ supply will render tissues hypoxic, which will cause them to release large amounts of lactic acid (resulting in metabolic acidosis). Respiration must be restored in a very few minutes if permanent damage to sensitive tissues is to be avoided.

A still more serious situation occurs in a cardiac arrest, in which all circulation of blood ceases. Each tissue becomes a closed system, its $O_2$ supply limited to that which was present in the tissue at the moment of arrest, and its $CO_2$ production forced to accumulate in the tissue. Again, the lessening $O_2$ supply will result in large amounts of lactic acid being released in tissues throughout the body. In this situation, however, the rapidly metabolizing tissues such as brain and heart cannot draw on the $O_2$ and nutrient reserves of the whole body, nor can their $CO_2$ production be poured into the body as a whole. Their metabolism therefore quickly ceases, and irreversible changes are wrought in the adult brain within 4–8 minutes. It is obvious that circulation and respiration must be quickly restored and maintained until cardiac function can be restored. The methods of choice are closed-chest cardiac massage and mouth-to-mouth ventilation. Even properly administered closed-chest cardiac massage, however, will deliver only about one-fifth of the normal resting cardiac output. This flow is sufficient to keep vital organs alive, but not enough to relieve the general tissue hypoxia, and the tissues therefore continue to generate lactic acid. Thus, $NaHCO_3$ must be administered periodically during the resuscitation to replace the $HCO_3^-$ destroyed by the lactic acid, so that the patient's acid–base status can be kept stable.

In some cases which require cardiopulmonary resuscitation (CPR), such as near drownings or near suffocation in a plastic bag, the CPR may itself bring about normal cardiac and respiratory function. In other cases such as sudden ventricular fibrillation, which is usually secondary to a heart attack, the CPR can be only a temporary measure to delay vital tissue death. Ventricular fibrillation never spontaneously reverts to normal cardiac function, but rather requires electrical defibrillation. It follows, therefore, that one of the first responsibilities of persons performing CPR is to contact competent emergency medical help and insure its prompt arrival at the scene.

## REFERENCES

1. Davenport, H. S. (1974): *The ABC of Acid-Base Chemistry,* 6th Ed. University of Chicago Press, Chicago.
2. Siggaard-Andersen, O. (1974): *The Acid-Base Status of the Blood,* 4th Ed. Williams and Wilkins, Baltimore.

## PROBLEMS

1. Points $X$ and $Y$ on Fig. 3 are values for blood samples taken from one of the following:

   a. a nervous candidate immediately before the final exam
   b. an individual addicted to TUMS (Antacid tablets)
   d. a normal person after 60 seconds of breath holding
   d. a patient arriving at the hospital in coma from a drug overdose of barbiturates
   e. a patient in diabetic coma (high blood content of acetoacetic and $\beta$-hydroxybutyric acid)

   A. What are values $X$ likely to be from?
   B. What are values $Y$ likely to be from?

2. Below is a list of arterial blood acid–base measurements:

   |     | pH | $P_{CO_2}$ (mm Hg) | $HCO_3^-$ (mEq/liter) | $P_{O_2}$ (mm Hg) |
   |-----|------|------|------|------|
   | a.  | 7.40 | 40 | 24 | 100 |
   | b.  | 7.61 | 20 | 19 | 40 |
   | c.  | 7.40 | 40 | 24 | 40 |
   | d.  | 7.21 | 80 | 32 | 100 |
   | e.  | 7.20 | 40 | 15 | 100 |

   A. Which of the above could be characterized as a pure respiratory alkalosis?
   B. Which of the above could be characterized as a pure respiratory acidosis?

3. A patient has complete pyloric obstruction for a day or two and has been vomiting all his gastric secretions including HCl and pepsin.

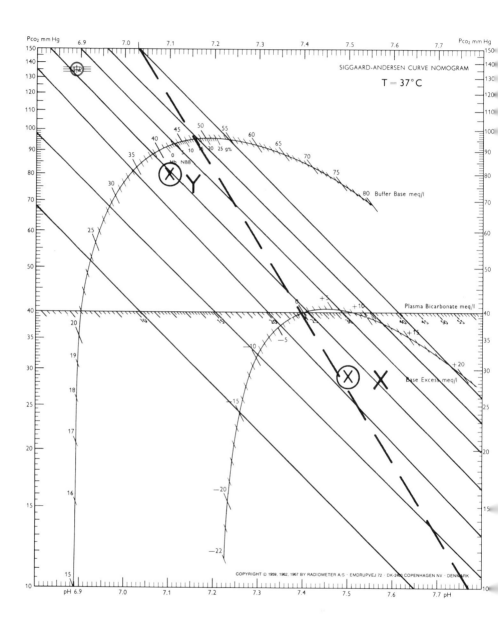

A. As a result of this, his arterial plasma would probably show
   a. abnormally high $P_{CO_2}$ and low or normal pH
   b. abnormally low $P_{CO_2}$ and high pH
   c. normal or high $P_{CO_2}$ and high pH
   d. abnormally high $P_{CO_2}$ and low $HCO_3^-$ concentration

B. His condition would best be termed
   a. respiratory acidosis
   b. respiratory alkalosis
   c. metabolic acidosis
   d. metabolic alkalosis
   e. normal acid–base status

4. A patient who has been suffering from diarrhea is found to have an arterial pH of 7.25 and an arterial $P_{CO_2}$ of 33 mm Hg.

  A. One would classify his condition as a primary
     a. respiratory acidosis
     b. respiratory alkalosis
     c. metabolic acidosis
     d. metabolic alkalosis
     c. normal acid–base status

  B. In the disturbance is of fairly recent onset, one would expect his oxyhemoglobin dissociation curve to be
     a. in its normal position
     b. shifted to the left
     c. shifted to the right
     d. shifted upward
     e. shifted downward

  C. One would expect his arterial
     a. plasma bicarbonate concentration to be higher than normal
     b. plasma bicarbonate concentration to be lower than normal
     c. plasma hydrogen ion concentration to be lower than normal
     d. plasma dissolved $CO_2$ concentration to be higher than normal
     e. blood buffer base to be higher than normal

5. Two subjects are identical and normal in every respect except that one is anemic and the other is polycythemic. If they both voluntarily hyperventilate by the same amount, in the new steady state the anemic subject will show

   a. the greater change in arterial total oxygen content
   b. the smaller change in percentage saturation of the arterial Hb

**FIG. 3.** A Siggaard-Andersen curve nomogram on which two samples of blood are plotted. (Reproduced with permission from *Radiometer*, Copenhagen.)

c. the greater change in alveolar carbon dioxide pressure
d. the smaller change in respiratory exchange ratio
e. the smaller change in arterial plasma bicarbonate concentration

6. A patient is brought into the hospital complaining of general weakness. He reports that he has been vomiting for several days. His arterial blood reveals that pH = 7.60, $Pa_{CO_2}$ = 40 mm Hg, and $Pa_{O_2}$ = 94 mm Hg. Decide which of the statements (a–f) are correct, and tell why you think so, and then answer question (g).

a. The patient has respiratory alkalosis (due to HCl being vomited).
b. The patient is probably ventilating at about a normal minute volume.
c. The patient has metabolic acidosis (due to $HCO_3^-$ being vomited).
d. The patient is probably hyperventilating.
e. The patient has metabolic alkalosis (due to HCl being vomited).
f. The patient is probably hypoxic.
g. What is the patient's arterial $HCO_3^-$ concentration?

7. A polio victim is brought into the hospital in the early stages of the disease one morning. He seems reasonably well that afternoon, but when he is tested the next morning (in obvious distress, breathless), his $PA_{CO_2}$ is 80 mm Hg, his $PA_{O_2}$ is 51 mm Hg, and his arterial pH is 7.20.

A. What is his arterial $HCO_3^-$ concentration?
B. The senior medical student in charge suggests an infusion of $NaHCO_3$ to correct the acidosis, and oxygen to relieve the hypoxia. Do you concur, or, if you don't agree, what is your choice of therapy, and why? Be sure to detail your treatment; in other words, tell how much $HCO_3^-$ you would give per kilogram body weight, or what inspired oxygen concentration you would use, or how much you would ventilate him with an artificial respirator, relative to his initial alveolar ventilation, or whether you would use continuous positive pressure ventilation, etc. Also, define his initial acid–base state (metabolic or respiratory acidosis or alkalosis).

## ANSWERS

1. **A:** Point $X$ is on the normal blood-buffer line at a $P_{CO_2}$ = 30 mm Hg. Thus, this is an acute respiratory alkalosis, which exists in many normal candidates immediately prior to a final exam. The answer is (a).
**B:** Point $Y$ has an extremely high $P_{CO_2}$ of 80 mm Hg, leading one to suspect very depressed breathing. The depressed breathing would also result in a very low $P_{O_2}$, which would cause the tissues to generate lactic acid, moving the point to the left of the normal blood–buffer line. The answer is (d).

2. **A:** Respiratory alkalosis must have a decreased $P_{CO_2}$; thus, the answer is (b).

**B:** Respiratory acidosis must have an elevated $P_{CO_2}$; thus, the answer is (d).

3. Vomiting HCl from the body will tend to cause a metabolic alkalosis in which the pH and $[HCO_3^-]$ will be high. The alkalosis may depress ventilation somewhat, which will elevate $CO_2$ somewhat. Thus, the answer for **A** is (c), and the answer for **B** is (d).

4. **A and C:** A person with diarrhea eliminates a fluid rich in $NaHCO_3$, thus inducing a metabolic acidosis with low pH and $[HCO_3^-]$. The blood acidity stimulates ventilation, lowering $P_{CO_2}$. Thus, the answer for **A** is (c), and the answer for **C** is (b).
   **B:** Acute acidosis shifts the Hb-$O_2$ dissociation curve to the right, but subsequent adjustments in 2,3-DPG tend to shift it back to where it was. Thus, early in the metabolic acidosis, the curve would be shifted to the right, and the answer is (c).

5. If two identical subjects hyperventilate identically, they will depress their alveolar carbon dioxide pressures identically, and will raise their alveolar oxygen pressures identically. The rise in oxygen pressure will dissolve extra amounts of oxygen identically, but the increased arterial saturation would mean more oxygen in the polycythemic subject, because he had more Hb, if anything. But since both subjects (presumably at sea level) are almost fully saturated anyway, the difference would be very small. The anemic subject, because his blood is less well buffered, would show the greater rise in arterial pH from the respiratory alkalosis. That would shift his Hb-$O_2$ dissociation curve to the left, which should favor, not impair, the saturation of his Hb. But the greater shift in pH for a given shift in $P_{CO_2}$ is equivalent to saying that there will be a smaller shift in bicarbonate concentration. Thus, the answer is (e).

6. a. NONSENSE.
   b. Since the $Pa_{CO_2}$ is about normal, the ventilation is about normal.
   c. NONSENSE
   d. Since the $Pa_{CO_2}$ is about normal, he is *not* hyperventilating.
   e. Alkalosis is present, but $PA_{CO_2} = 40$ mm Hg, therefore metabolic.
   f. $Pa_{O_2}$ is normal, therefore no evidence of hypoxia.
   g. The patient has an arterial $HCO_3^-$ concentration of 38 mEq/liter.

   $$pH = pK' + \log [HCO_3^-] - \log (0.03\ P_{CO_2});\ \log [HCO_3^-] = pH - pK' + \log (0.03\ P_{CO_2});\ \therefore [HCO_3^-] = 10^{(pH-pK)} (0.03\ P_{CO_2})$$

7. **A:** His arterial $HCO_3^-$ concentration is 30.2 mEq/liter.
   **B:** You simply need to increase ventilation to normal. Everything else will then also return to normal. Respiratory acidosis must be corrected by adjusting effective ventilation.

# 7

## Gas Exchange in the Lungs

In Chapter 3 we discussed how ventilation brings environmental gas into the alveoli and alveolar gas back out to the environment through convection. The linear velocity of that flow is quite high in the upper airways, but gets slower and slower as the airways branch and their cross-sectional area thus increases. Between the trachea and the terminal branchings of the respiratory tree, the alveolar ducts, the cross-sectional area has increased by a factor of almost 5,000. Thus, while the linear velocity of gas molecules in the trachea may be 200 cm/sec during quiet inspiration, it will be only about 0.4 mm/sec through the alveolar ducts in quiet inspiration. The velocity of flow will be much slower than this in the alveoli themselves, and will be quite ineffective in moving gas between alveolar duct and alveolar surface. Fortunately, over these small distances, gas diffusion is quite capable of effecting the exchange between the alveolar ducts and the alveolar surfaces. Diffusion of the respiratory gases through liquids and tissues must then effect exchange between alveolar surfaces and erythrocytes.

This chapter begins with a consideration of gas diffusion, first through a gas phase and then through a liquid phase. Next there is a brief coverage of the theory behind the measurement of diffusing capacity of the lung and a word or two about practical methods used in that measurement. A discussion of ventilation–perfusion relationships in the lung follows, with some semiquantitative models as examples. Finally, right-to-left (R–L) shunts are discussed, again using semiquantitative examples.

### DIFFUSION—GASES IN GASES

The molecules of gases are in constant motion. If the concentration of the molecules of a given gas is greater in one region than in another, this constant movement will tend to cause diffusion from the region of higher concentration to that of the lower, and will tend to equalize the concentrations of the gas in the two regions. This process occurs because, statistically, more molecules of the gas move from the region of higher concentration to the region of lower concentration than the reverse.

Under similar conditions of temperature and pressure, different gases have the same translational energy. Thus, ½ (mv²) for one gas equals ½ (mv²) for any other, under the same conditions of T and P. It is intuitively obvious, therefore, that heavier gas molecules will move more slowly and diffuse more slowly than lighter ones. It is easy to quantitate this relationship: $mv^2 = m'$ $(v')^2$, or $v^2/(v')^2 = m'/m$, or $v/v' = \sqrt{m'/m}$. Thus, the ratio of the rates of diffusion of two gases (through gas) will be inversely proportional to the ratios of their molecular weights. This relationship, called Graham's law, can be used to show that $CO_2$ diffuses 85% as rapidly as $O_2$ through gas phase under the same conditions of P and T:

$$\frac{\text{Rate for } CO_2}{\text{Rate for } O_2} = \frac{\sqrt{MW\ O_2}}{\sqrt{MW\ CO_2}} = \frac{\sqrt{32}}{\sqrt{44}} = \frac{5.6}{6.6} = 0.85$$

Thus, $CO_2$ and $O_2$ diffuse at roughly similar rates through alveolar gas. How adequate are those rates? How quickly will fresh environmental gas which has been brought to the alveoli come into equilibrium with the alveolar gas already present? Comroe has estimated that, even if the diffusion distance were 0.5 mm, diffusion of the $O_2$ and $CO_2$ would be 80% complete in 0.002 seconds. Since the average alveolar diameter is only about 0.1 mm, it is clear that any difference between the concentration of a gas in one part of a normal alveolus and that in another part would be eliminated in a small fraction of a second. Thus, diffusion of gases within gases poses no problem for the normal lung. However, if alveolar diameters (and therefore diffusion distances) become orders of magnitude greater, as occurs in emphysema (in which alveolar septa are destroyed), then $Po_2$ and $Pco_2$ may not be the same throughout each alveolus.

## DIFFUSION—GASES IN LIQUIDS

Diffusion through a gas phase is responsible for exchange of gases between alveolar duct and alveolar surface, but diffusion through liquid phases must occur to effect the exchange between alveolar surface and red blood cells. An $O_2$ molecule passing from the gas phase at the alveolar surface to a hemoglobin molecule in an erythrocyte would have to pass through the following structures (seen in Fig. 1): (a) the surfactant layer, (b) the alveolar epithelial cell (involving two cell membranes and cell cytoplasm), (c) a basement membrane, (d) a capillary endothelial cell (again involving two cell membranes surrounding cell cytoplasm), (e) plasma, and (f) the erythrocyte membrane. The total thickness of this aggregate liquid barrier (at regions where cell nuclei are not present) is less than a micron.

The rate at which a gas diffuses through liquid phases depends both on Graham's law (as just discussed), and on the solubility of the gas in the liquid. This latter factor is important because the diffusion of a gas really depends on its concentration difference. In a gas phase, the concentration of a gas is

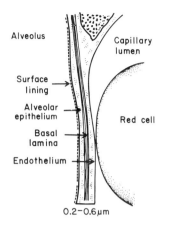

Alveolus

Capillary lumen

Surface lining

Alveolar epithelium

Red cell

Basal lamina

Endothelium

0.2–0.6μm

**FIG. 1.** The alveolar capillary membranes. To reach the red cell, $O_2$ traverses the surface lining layer, the alveolar epithelial cytoplasm, the basal lamina, the endothelial cell cytoplasm, and the plasma. In some locations, there is also loose interstitial tissue between the epithelium and the endothelium. (Approximate magnification ×20,000.) (Reproduced with permission from Ganong, W. F., *Review of Medical Physiology*, 8th Ed., Lange Medical Publications, Los Altos, CA, 1977.)

directly proportional to the partial pressure alone. In a liquid phase, the concentration of the molecules of a given gas is directly proportional to the partial pressure of that gas times its solubility in that liquid. For a given partial pressure difference across a liquid barrier, therefore, an extremely soluble gas will have a much greater concentration difference than a rather insoluble gas, and will tend to diffuse far more easily. Henry's law, which permits one to calculate the concentration of gas in liquid, knowing its partial pressure and solubility, is symbolized thus: Concentration of gas $X$ in a given liquid $= P_X(\alpha)$, where $P_X$ is the partial pressure of gas $X$ and $\alpha$ is its solubility coefficient. For $O_2$ in watery solutions, $\alpha$ is about (0.03 ml $O_2$/liter fluid)/mm Hg. For $CO_2$ in watery solutions, $\alpha$ is about (0.7 ml $CO_2$/liter fluid)/mm Hg. Thus, $CO_2$ is some *23 times as soluble as is $O_2$ in the watery phases* through which they must both diffuse between alveolar gas and the red blood cells. To compare the diffusibility of $CO_2$ and $O_2$ through water phases, then, requires a combination of Graham's and Henry's laws, namely:

$$\frac{\text{Diffusibility of } CO_2}{\text{Diffusibility of } O_2} = \frac{5.6}{6.6} \times 23 = \text{about } \frac{20}{1}$$

$CO_2$ thus diffuses 20 times as easily as $O_2$ through water phases, whereas it diffuses only 0.85 times as easily as $O_2$ through gas phases.

## DIFFUSION OF $O_2$ AND $CO_2$ BETWEEN ALVEOLAR GAS AND BLOOD

At rest, blood normally spends about 0.75 seconds in pulmonary capillaries exposed to alveolar gas. We can follow the time course of the changes in partial pressures of $O_2$ and $CO_2$ in that capillary blood, as seen in Fig. 2. Here, the ordinate is both $P_{O_2}$ and $P_{CO_2}$, calibrated in mm Hg, and extending over the range bracketed by mixed venous blood on the one hand and alveolar gas on the other. We simplify the situation by pretending that the alveolar gas $P_{O_2}$

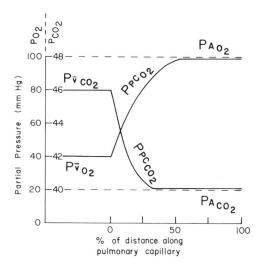

**FIG. 2.** $P_{O_2}$ and $P_{CO_2}$ of pulmonary capillary blood before and during its exposure to alveolar gas. The alveolar $P_{O_2}$ **(Top)** and the alveolar $P_{CO_2}$ **(bottom)** are presumed unchanging at their normal mean values and are indicated by *dashed lines.*

and $P_{CO_2}$ are constant (remember, they really vary by 1 or 2 mm Hg from one part of the respiratory cycle to another) at 100 and 40 mm Hg, respectively (dashed lines). The mixed venous blood (solid lines) arrives at the alveoli having a $P_{O_2}$ of about 40 mm Hg and a $P_{CO_2}$ of about 46 mm Hg. Thus, there is initially a huge partial pressure difference for $O_2$ from alveolar gas. Diffusion of the two gases along their concentration differences proceeds, and the respective partial pressures in the blood approach those in the alveolar gas, reaching equilibrium with it long before the blood leaves the alveoli. In fact, within 0.3 seconds for $O_2$, and sooner for $CO_2$, equilibration is achieved. $CO_2$ is able to achieve equilibration sooner even though it has a lesser partial pressure difference driving it, because it diffuses about 20 times as easily as does $O_2$. In exercise, the blood flow increases greatly, and each red cell may spend much less than 0.75 seconds in the alveoli, but never in health or during normal activity is the time less than the 0.3 seconds needed for equilibration. If the alveolar membranes thicken greatly, gas diffusion can be impeded enough so that $O_2$ never reaches equilibration between alveolar gas and pulmonary capillary blood, but it takes a combination of severe exercise (to decrease residence time of blood in pulmonary capillaries) and hypoxia (to decrease the driving $P_{O_2}$ from alveolar gas to pulmonary capillary blood) to accomplish this. Carbon dioxide, on the other hand, essentially always achieves equilibration between alveolar gas and blood, because of its much greater diffusibility.

## MEASUREMENT OF PULMONARY DIFFUSING CAPACITY

The flow of a given gas across a barrier can be quantified generally thus:

$$\dot{V} = (d)(A/T)(P_1 - P_2)$$

where $\dot{V}$ is the volume flow of the gas in ml/min, d is a constant describing the diffusibility of that gas in the material of that barrier and incorporating both Graham's law and Henry's law, A is the area available for diffusion, T is the thickness of the barrier, and $P_1$ and $P_2$ are the partial pressures of that gas on either side of the barrier. In a simple model system, it may be possible to measure the values of A and T accurately, but it is not easy in the lung. For this reason, d is usually combined with A and T to yield a diffusion constant for the lung, $DL$. The rearranged equation then looks like this:

$$DL = \dot{V}/(P_1 - P_2)$$

where $DL$ has the units (ml/min)/mm Hg.

To characterize the diffusing capacity of a given lung for $O_2$, then, one must measure $\dot{V}O_2$, $PA_{O_2}$, and $Ppc_{O_2}$. The problem is that $Ppc_{O_2}$ changes all along the course of the pulmonary capillary, beginning at the mixed venous level and finally reaching equilibrium with the alveolar $PO_2$. To measure $DL_{O_2}$, then, requires the calculation of an integrated mean pulmonary capillary $PO_2$, which can be done through the use of a formula and some assumptions.

The same information can be gleaned, however, and far more easily, through the measurement of the diffusing capacity of the lung for carbon monoxide. CO, supplied to the alveolar gas, follows the same diffusion pathway as $O_2$, and binds to the same site on the Hb molecules. The advantages of this gas are twofold: (a) the gas is normally in very low concentration in the environment (except in the case of smokers) and thus there is essentially none in the mixed venous blood coming into the lungs; and (b) the affinity of CO for Hb is 210 times that of $O_2$, so that any molecules of CO which pass from alveolar gas to blood are immediately bound tightly to Hb, and therefore the partial pressure of CO stays essentially zero in the pulmonary capillary blood. Of course, very low concentrations of CO (e.g., 0.3%) are employed, and even those for only a short time. The equation then becomes: $DL_{CO} = \dot{V}CO/PA_{CO}$, and one needs only to measure the uptake of CO and the alveolar $PCO$ to make the calculation. Fortunately, it is possible to combine Graham's and Henry's laws again to compare the diffusibility of $O_2$ and CO through the membranes of the lung. Thus:

$$\frac{DL_{O_2}}{DL_{CO}} = \frac{\text{Solubility } O_2}{\text{Solubility CO}} \times \frac{\sqrt{MW_{CO}}}{\sqrt{MW_{O_2}}} = 1.25$$

Thus, $DL_{O_2} = 1.25\ (DL_{CO})$, and $DL_{O_2}$ can be calculated, although $DL_{CO}$ has been measured for the reasons stated above.

Practically speaking, there are several ways to measure $DL_{CO}$, the simplest of which is the single-breath test. Here, the patient inspires a gas mixture containing a low percentage of CO, then holds his breath for 10 seconds. The $\dot{V}CO$ can be calculated from the percentage of CO in the alveolar gas at the beginning and end of the 10-second period, if one also knows the volume of the alveolar gas. $PA_{CO}$, which is the only other piece of information needed, varies during the 10-second period as CO moves from alveolar gas to pulmonary capillary blood, but its mean value can be calculated.

Normal values (in a healthy, normal-sized adult at rest) are (25 ml/min)/ mm Hg for $DL_{CO}$ and, by calculation, (31 ml/min)/mm Hg for $DL_{O_2}$. It should be realized that these normal resting values increase markedly during exercise, probably because the area for diffusion increases as more pulmonary capillaries open and/or because those already open open more widely.

## VENTILATION/PERFUSION RELATIONSHIPS AND R–L SHUNTS

The last few paragraphs have emphasized that equilibration for both $PO_2$ and $PCO_2$ normally occurs between gas and blood in each alveolus. Nevertheless, normally, the blood that has been returned to the left heart via the pulmonary veins and pumped out to the systemic arteries has a markedly lower $PO_2$ than does the mixed alveolar gas. That is, arterial $PO_2$ ($Pa_{O_2}$) may be only about 90 mm Hg, while alveolar gas or end-tidal gas $PO_2$ ($PA_{O_2}$) may be about 100 mm Hg. This difference arises because, even in normal people (a) there exists mismatching of ventilation and blood flow among the alveoli, and (b) there exists some small percentage of the body's venous return which bypasses the gas exchange process in the lungs, thereby becoming an R-L shunt (venous admixture).

## VENTILATION–PERFUSION MISMATCHING

Both lungs together receive a total of about 4 liters/min of alveolar ventilation ($\dot{V}A$) and about 5 liters/min of blood flow ($\dot{Q}$), for an overall $\dot{V}A/\dot{Q}$ ratio of about 0.8. Because of gravity, however, upright man's $\dot{V}A/\dot{Q}$ ratios vary greatly from one part of the lungs to another.

The blood flow or perfusion to the apex of the lung is very much less than that to the base (by a factor of about six). This occurs because the pulmonary artery pressure is rather low relative to the columns of blood that exist in the lung, and because the lung vessels are collapsible and distensible. The lung may be 40 cm long in a tall person, and the hilum, where the pulmonary arteries enter and the pulmonary veins leave the lung, is about at the midpoint of that 40 cm. Thus, gravity adds about 20 cm $H_2O$ to the intravascular pressure at the base of the lungs, and subtracts about 20 cm $H_2O$ from the intravascular pressure at the apex. The pulmonary artery pressure (just past the tricuspid valve) may be only 25/8 mm Hg, which converts to 34/11 cm $H_2O$. Thus, at least during diastole, the intravascular pressure at the apex of the lung will become subatmospheric by 9 cm $H_2O$. The extravascular pressure is closely related to the alveolar pressure, which fluctuates 1 or 2 cm $H_2O$ above and 1 or 2 cm $H_2O$ below atmospheric during normal breathing. So, during diastole, the intravascular pressure become less than the extravascular pressure at the apex of the lung causing vessels to collapse and flow to stop. (Positive pressure respiration might raise the alveolar pressure enough to close vessels at the apex of the lung throughout the cardiac cycle.) Even the zones of the lung lower down, in which all intravascular pressures are greater than alveolar pressure, are affected by the gravitational field. Here, the pressure added to the arteries by gravity is exactly equal to the pressure added to the veins, and the driving pressures are thus unaffected. The transmural pressure of all vessels is increased, however, by about 20 cm $H_2O$, at the base of the lung. This dilates these vessels, lowering their resistance to flow, so that more flow occurs even with unchanged driving pressure.

The alveolar ventilation is also less to the apex of the lung than it is to the base, but the factor is only about 2.5. Gravity is again responsible, causing the intrapleural pressure to be more subatmospheric at the apex of the lung than at the base. This occurs because the lungs "hang," as it were, in the pleural cavity, and their weight tends to pull them away from the apex of that cavity rather strongly, making the intrapleural pressure at the apex quite subatmospheric. Further down the lung, there is less weight "pulling," contributing less "suction;" and at the bases of the lung, the intrapleural pressure may be only just subatmospheric. Thus, although students are given the figure of about −5 cm $H_2O$ as a "normal" intrapleural pressure, they must realize that there is a whole spectrum of intrapleural pressures. At functional residual capacity (FRC) in upright people, for instance, the intrapleural pressure at the apices of the lung may be −10 cm $H_2O$ while it is −2.5 cm $H_2O$ at the bases. Because of this difference in intrapleural pressures, there exists a difference in transpulmonary pressures, and the apical alveoli are expanded much more than the basal ones at FRC. Figure 3 shows a normal plot of the percentage of total lung capacity versus transpulmonary pressure. The curve has an initial steep slope, followed by a less steep but reasonably linear middle segment, and finally its

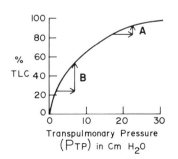

FIG. 3. Lung volume vs transpulmonary pressure (PTP), showing the volume increment caused by increasing the PTP by 5 cm $H_2O$ at each of two initial volumes. At *A*, lung is on stiffer part of compliance range and volume increment is less than at *B* where compliance is greater. During a breath from FRC, apical alveoli change volume as at *A*, while those nearer the base change volume as at *B*.

slope decreases again, approaching zero as lung volume approaches 100% total lung capacity (TLC). Since this slope, $\Delta V/\Delta P$, is the lung compliance, this means that the lung compliance is initially great, is lesser but linear in the midrange, and finally is lesser and lesser approaching zero at TLC. This curve describes the behavior of the lung as a whole, but we have just concluded that at FRC, the apical alveoli are very much more expanded than are the basal ones. During a breath from FRC, therefore, the apical alveoli may operate on the stiff part of their compliance curve, while the basal ones are much more compliant. Thus, a given change in transpulmonary pressure of 5 cm $H_2O$ will cause a larger change in volume of the basal alveoli (B) than in the apical alveoli (A).

So, perfusion ($\dot{Q}$) is 6 times higher at the bases of the lung than it is at the apex, and alveolar ventilation ($\dot{V}A$) is about 2.5 times greater at the base of the lung than it is at the apex. The $\dot{V}A/\dot{Q}$ ratio, then, is 6/2.5 or about 2.4 times greater at the apex than at the base. Let us consider the $\dot{V}A/\dot{Q}$ continuum in Fig. 4 to get an idea of the implications of this normal situation. The line marked $A$ in Fig. 4 is the $\dot{V}A/\dot{Q}$ continuum, and shows those ratios from the one theoretically possible extreme to the other. Thus, a $\dot{V}A/\dot{Q}$ ratio of zero would mean that there was no $\dot{V}A$ to a part of the lung that was still being perfused with blood, and $\dot{V}A/\dot{Q}$ ratio of infinity would mean that there was no perfusion to a part of the lung that was still being ventilated. The $\dot{V}A/\dot{Q}$ ratio of 0.8 in the center of this continuum is the "ideal" ratio that would exist in all alveoli if the total $\dot{V}A$ of 4 liters/min and the total $\dot{Q}$ of about 5 liters/min were to be evenly apportioned among all the alveoli.

The drawings marked $B$ are meant to illustrate these three $\dot{V}A/\dot{Q}$ ratios. The drawing over the $\dot{V}A/\dot{Q}$ ratio of zero shows blood flow occuring without alveolar ventilation. This blood flow would pass unchanged from the right heart through the lungs to the left heart, and therefore would be the equivalent of a R–L shunt. Fortunately, there are no alveoli with $\dot{V}A/\dot{Q}$ ratios less than about 0.5–0.6 in normal lungs. The other theoretically possible extreme is depicted over the continuum at the $\dot{V}A/\dot{Q}$ ratio of infinity. These alveoli would be ventilated while receiving no blood flow. This alveolar ventilation, like the

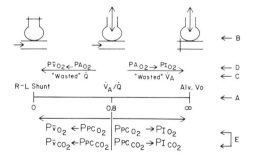

**FIG. 4.** Various aspects of the $\dot{V}A/\dot{Q}$ continuum.

anatomic dead space ventilation, would be ineffective in gas exchange and thus would ventilate what has been called the "alveolar dead space." Again fortunately, there are no such alveoli in normal lungs, the highest $\dot{V}A/\dot{Q}$ ratios found being 2–2.5. The situation depicted over the $\dot{V}A/\dot{Q}$ ratio of 0.8 is the one in which alveolar ventilation is nicely matched to blood flow.

Thus, although there are no alveoli that have $\dot{V}A/\dot{Q}$ ratios anywhere near either theoretical limit in normal lungs, there are alveoli whose ratios lie to either side of the "ideal" ratio of 0.8. The arrows marked $C$ in Fig. 4 provide a useful way to view these two groups of alveoli. Those alveoli to the right of (at higher $\dot{V}A/\dot{Q}$ ratios than) the "ideal" of 0.8 have too much ventilation in relation to their blood flow; thus, some of their alveolar ventilation is "wasted." Those alveoli to the left of (at lower $\dot{V}A/\dot{Q}$ ratios than) the "ideal" of 0.8 have too much blood flow in relation to their alveolar ventilation; thus, some of their blood flow is "wasted."

The information marked $D$ in Fig. 4 shows the direction in which $PA_{O_2}$ would be expected to change in alveoli with ratios above and below the ideal $\dot{V}A/\dot{Q}$ ratio of 0.8. It is again useful to consider the theoretically possible extremes first. At a $\dot{V}A/\dot{Q}$ ratio of infinity, there is no blood flow to remove $O_2$ from or add $CO_2$ to the inspired gas; $PI_{O_2}$ and $PI_{CO_2}$ would therefore remain unchanged in these alveoli. It should be intuitively obvious, then, that the $PA_{O_2}$ (and $PA_{CO_2}$) of alveoli whose $\dot{V}A/\dot{Q}$ ratios are greater than 0.8 approach the $PO_2$ (and $PCO_2$) of the inspired gas as their $\dot{V}A/\dot{Q}$ ratio approaches infinity. Since the ideal alveoli at sea level have a $PA_{O_2}$ of about 100 mm Hg and a $PA_{CO_2}$ of about 40 mm Hg, these alveoli would have $PA_{O_2} > 100$ mm Hg and $PA_{CO_2} < 40$ mm Hg. Conversely, alveoli with a $\dot{V}A/\dot{Q}$ ratio of zero would have no ventilation to add $O_2$ to or remove $CO_2$ from their blood flow. The mixed venous gas pressures ($P\bar{v}_{O_2}$ and $P\bar{v}_{CO_2}$) would therefore remain unchanged as blood passes through these alveoli. It should be intuitively obvious that the $PA_{O_2}$ and $PA_{CO_2}$ of these poorly ventilated alveoli should approach those of the mixed venous blood as their $\dot{V}A/\dot{Q}$ ratios approach zero. Their $PA_{O_2}$ would be $< 100$ mm Hg and their $PA_{CO_2}$ would be $> 40$ mm Hg.

We already know that the $PO_2$ and $PCO_2$ of the pulmonary capillary blood of any given alveolus reaches equilibrium with its $PA_{O_2}$ and $PA_{CO_2}$. Therefore, as shown in Fig. 4E, the pulmonary capillary partial pressures of those alveoli to the right of a $\dot{V}A/\dot{Q}$ ratio of 0.8 approach those of the inspired gas ($Ppc_{O_2}{\rightarrow}{\rightarrow}{\rightarrow}PI_{O_2}$, and $Ppc_{CO_2}{\rightarrow}{\rightarrow}{\rightarrow}PI_{CO_2}$) as the $\dot{V}A/\dot{Q}$ ratio approaches infinity. Similarly, in those alveoli with $\dot{V}A/\dot{Q}$ ratios less than 0.8, $Ppc_{O_2}$ and $Ppc_{CO_2}$ approach $P\bar{v}_{O_2}$ and $P\bar{v}_{CO_2}$, respectively, as the $\dot{V}A/\dot{Q}$ ratio approaches zero.

## EFFECT OF ALVEOLI WITH $\dot{V}A/\dot{Q}$ RATIOS HIGHER AND LOWER THAN 0.8 ON ARTERIAL $PO_2$ AND $PCO_2$

Let us first consider a simple if somewhat unrealistic lung model which has some of its alveoli with $\dot{V}A/\dot{Q}$ ratios higher than 0.8, and the rest of its alveoli with $\dot{V}_A/\dot{Q}$ ratios lower than 0.8. Further, let 2 liters/min of alveolar ventilation go to each group of alveoli, and set the $\dot{V}_A/\dot{Q}$ ratios such that the first group of alveoli has a $P_{A_{O_2}}$ of 140 mm Hg and the second has a $P_{A_{O_2}}$ of 60 mm Hg.

It is easy to see that 2 liters/min of alveolar gas with a $P_{O_2}$ of 60 mm Hg mixing with 2 liters/min of alveolar gas having a $P_{O_2}$ of 140 mm Hg will give 4 liters/min of mixed alveolar gas whose $P_{O_2}$ is a nice normal value of 100 mm Hg.

It is not so easy to see that the mixed pulmonary venous $P_{O_2}$ will be less than 100 mm Hg, but it is true, and there are two main reasons for it. The first reason involves the sigmoid shape of the Hb-$O_2$ dissociation curve, as pictured in Fig. 5. Simply stated, the shape of the curve is such that the blood perfusing the high $\dot{V}_A/\dot{Q}$ alveoli will have little extra $O_2$ content, while the blood perfusing the low $\dot{V}_A/\dot{Q}$ alveoli will have significantly less $O_2$ content than normal. The blood coming into equilibrium with the $P_{A_{O_2}}$ of 60 mm Hg (low $\dot{V}_A/\dot{Q}$) will have an $O_2$ content of 181 ml/liter blood, while that coming into equilibrium with the $P_{A_{O_2}}$ of 140 mm Hg (high $\dot{V}_A/\dot{Q}$) will have an $O_2$ content of 199 ml/liter blood. These two streams of blood will mix in the pulmonary veins. If there were equal flows of blood perfusing these two groups of alveoli, then the $O_2$ content of the mixed pulmonary venous blood would be halfway between the contents of the two streams, or 190 ml/liter blood. Under these conditions the $P_{O_2}$ of the mixed pulmonary venous blood would be about 79 mm Hg, quite far from the mixed alveolar $P_{O_2}$ of 100 mm Hg.

But the situation is far worse than this for the second reason, which is that most of the blood flow will come from the low $\dot{V}_A/\dot{Q}$ regions. In the obviously

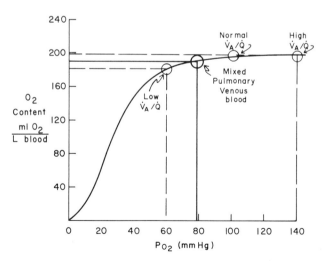

**FIG. 5.** Low blood $P_{O_2}$ caused by the mixing of equal flows of blood from high and low $\dot{V}_A/Q$ ratios.

exaggerated example we have chosen, 29/30 of the flow would come from the alveoli with the $P_{O_2}$ of 60 mm Hg, and only 1/30 would come from the alveoli with the $P_{O_2}$ of 140 mm Hg. Thus, the actual content of the mixed pulmonary venous blood would be weighted very heavily toward the low $\dot{V}_A/\dot{Q}$ alveoli, and will be actually 181.6 ml/liter blood, which will correspond to a $P_{O_2}$ of 61 or 62 mm Hg. Thus, in our example, the $P_{O_2}$ of the mixed pulmonary capillary blood will be *very* far from the $P_{O_2}$ of the mixed alveolar gas (62 versus 100), even though the gas and blood of each alveolus reach equilibrium with one another.

Much smaller differences between $P_{CO_2}$ of mixed alveolar and mixed pulmonary venous blood develop as a result of $\dot{V}_A/\dot{Q}$ mismatching, largely because the $CO_2$ content of high $\dot{V}_A/\dot{Q}$ alveoli tends to cancel out the high $CO_2$ content in low $\dot{V}_A/\dot{Q}$ alveoli. What differences there are between mixed alveolar gas and mixed pulmonary venous blood develop because of the second reason (above) which weights the mixed pulmonary blood content strongly toward the content of the low $\dot{V}_A/\dot{Q}$ alveoli. These differences tend to be small also because the $CO_2$ dissociation curve is so much steeper than is the Hb-$O_2$ dissociation curve. That is, moderately large changes in $CO_2$ content of blood can occur without changing the $P_{CO_2}$ by more than a few millimeters of mercury.

Now let us consider the more reasonable three-compartment model of the lung shown in Fig. 6. Here, we have an overall $\dot{V}_A = 4$ liters/min, and an overall $\dot{Q} = 5$ liters/min, for an overall $\dot{V}_A/\dot{Q}$ ratio of 0.8, all normal values. These $\dot{V}_A$ and $\dot{Q}$ have been apportioned to the three compartments much as they might be in an upright person, such that the $\dot{V}_A/\dot{Q}$ ratio is high at the apex (2.0), lower in the middle (1.2), and lowest at the base (0.5). The $P_{A_{O_2}}$ have been chosen appropriate to the $\dot{V}_A/\dot{Q}$ ratios, being 120 at the apex, 110 in the middle, and 87 at the base, for a mixed $P_{A_{O_2}}$ of 102 mm Hg: $[1(120) + 1.2(110) + 1.8(87)]/4 = 102$ mm Hg.

To calculate the $P_{O_2}$ of the mixed pulmonary venous blood, we must first find the $O_2$ content of that blood after the streams coming from the three compartments have mixed. (We can then look up the $P_{O_2}$ on an Hb-$O_2$ dissociation curve). To do that requires (a) determining the $O_2$ content per liter of blood of each stream, (b) multiplying that by the flow rate in liters of blood

| Compart-ments | $\dot{V}_A$ | $\dot{Q}$ | $\dot{V}_A/\dot{Q}$ | $P_{A_{O_2}}$ |
|---|---|---|---|---|
| I | 1.0 | 0.5 | 2.0 | 120 |
| II | 1.2 | 1.0 | 1.2 | 110 |
| III | 1.8 | 3.5 | 0.5 | 87 |

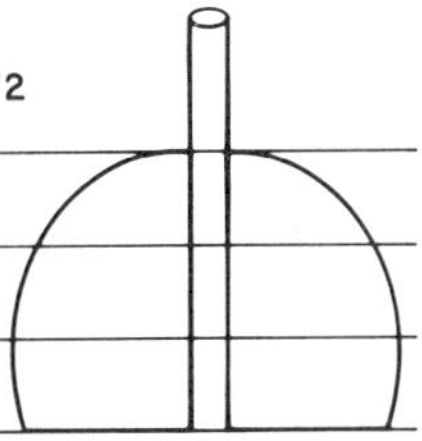

**FIG. 6.** A three-compartment model of the lung with values of $\dot{V}_A$, $\dot{Q}$, $\dot{V}_A/\dot{Q}$ ratio, and $P_{A_{O_2}}$ which are reasonably normal overall.

per minute in that stream ($\dot{Q}$) to get the amount of $O_2$ delivered per minute by that stream to the mixed pulmonary blood, (c) dividing the total amount of $O_2$ brought to the mixed pulmonary venous blood by the total amount of blood which brings it, to get the $O_2$ content of the mixed blood. The worksheet in Fig. 7 is meant to aid in this series of calculations. In category 1 (vertical column 1) are listed the $PA_{O_2}$ of each of the three compartments, and the mixed alveolar $P_{O_2}$ at the bottom; this was calculated as described above using the $\dot{V}A$ of the individual compartments and the overall or total $\dot{V}A$ as given in category 2. The $\dot{Q}$ of the individual compartments and their total are listed in category 6. Thus, category 12 shows the results of dividing the $\dot{V}A$ in category 2 by the $\dot{Q}$ in category 6 to get the $\dot{V}A/\dot{Q}$ ratios of the individual compartments and the $\dot{V}A/\dot{Q}$ ratio overall.

Next, using the $PA_{O_2}$ of each compartment and assuming that there is equilibrium between $P_{O_2}$ of alveolar gas and pulmonary capillary blood, we need to look up the $O_2$ content of each liter of blood draining from each of the three compartments. Row A of the tabulated data on the lower left of Fig. 7 gives those $O_2$ contents for any $P_{O_2}$ from 10 to 140 mm Hg; rows B, C, and D give additional information about, respectively, how much of that content is dissolved, how much is bound to Hb, and what the percent saturation of the Hb is at $P_{O_2}$ values from 10 to 140 mm Hg. The reader is invited to fill in categories 3 and 4 with the data in rows B and C of the tabulated data, but all that is really needed is to fill in category 5 with the data from row A. So, compartment I, which has an alveolar $P_{O_2} = 120$ mm Hg, will have an $O_2$ content of 197 ml/liter blood. Compartments II and III, with $PA_{O_2}$ of 110 and 87, will have $O_2$ contents of 196 and 194 ml/liter blood, respectively. We now know how much $O_2$ is brought to the pulmonary veins in each liter of blood draining from each of the three compartments. To find the total amount of $O_2$ draining from each compartment, we need to multiply its $O_2$ content/liter blood by its $\dot{Q}$ in liters per minute. Thus, multiplying the data in category 5 by that in category 6 in each case, we get 98.5, 196, and 679 ml $O_2$/min from compartments I, II, and III, respectively, for a total delivery of $O_2$ to the pulmonary veins of 973.5 ml $O_2$/min. When the blood in these three streams has mixed, that 973.5 ml $O_2$/min will be distributed evenly in the total $\dot{Q}$ of 5 liters/min; thus, in category 8, we find that there will be 194.7 ml $O_2$ in each of those 5 liters. Looking back along row A of the table at the lower left, we see that blood will have 194 ml $O_2$/liters when its $P_{O_2}$ is 90 mm Hg and 195 ml $O_2$/liter when its $P_{O_2}$ is 100 mm Hg. Since this blood has 194.7 ml $O_2$/liter, its $P_{O_2}$ must be about two-thirds of the way from 90 to 100, and I have listed it as 97 mm Hg at the bottom of category 10. To fill in category 9, interpolate similarly along row D of the table.

The relevance of this calculation becomes clear when one compares the figure at the bottom of category 1 with that at the bottom of category 10. Even though there was perfect equilibrium for $P_{O_2}$ between alveolar gas and pulmonary capillary blood in each of the three compartments of this model lung, there is a

CATEGORIES

| | 1 | 2 | 3 | 4 | 5 | 6 | 7 | 8 | 9 | 10 | 11 | 12 |
|---|---|---|---|---|---|---|---|---|---|---|---|---|
| COMPARTMENT | $P_{A}O_2$ mm Hg | $\dot{V}_A$ liter/min | $[O_2]$ as $[HbO_2]$ ml/liter | $[O_2]$diss. ml/liter | (3) + (4) ml/liter | $\dot{Q}$ liter/min | (5) × (6) ml $O_2$/min | Total $O_2$ Carried By Blood | Mixed Blood % Sat. | Mixed Blood $PO_2$ (mm Hg) | Gas – Bl $\Delta PO_2$ (mm Hg) | $\dot{V}_A/\dot{Q}$ |
| I | 120 | 1.0 | 193 | 4 | 197 | 0.5 | 98.5 | | | | | 2.0 |
| II | 110 | 1.2 | 193 | 3 | 196 | 1.0 | 196 | | | | | 1.2 |
| III | 87 | 1.8 | 191 | 3 | 194 | 3.5 | 679 | | | | | 0.5 |
| IV TOTALS, MEANS, MIXED GAS, BL | Mean $P_{A}O_2$ 102 | Total $\dot{V}_A$ 4.0 | | | | Total $\dot{Q}$ 5.0 | 973.5 | $[O_2]$ of Mixed Blood (ml/liter) 194.7 | 97.3 | 97 | 5 | Overall $\dot{V}_A/\dot{Q}$ 0.8 |

**A** WHOLE BLOOD $[O_2]$ ml $O_2$/liter blood

| 199 | 197 | 195 | 194 | 191 | 187 | 181 | 169 | 148 | 114 | 64.4 | 19.2 |
|---|---|---|---|---|---|---|---|---|---|---|---|

**B** DISSOLVED $[O_2]$ ml $O_2$/liter blood

| 4.2 | 3.6 | 3.0 | 2.7 | 2.4 | 2.1 | 1.8 | 1.5 | 1.2 | 0.9 | 0.6 | 0.3 |
|---|---|---|---|---|---|---|---|---|---|---|---|

**C** $[O_2]$ combined with Hb ml $O_2$/liter blood

| 194 | 193 | 192 | 191 | 189 | 185 | 179 | 168 | 147 | 113 | 63.8 | 18.9 |
|---|---|---|---|---|---|---|---|---|---|---|---|

**D** % Saturation of Hb $(HbO_2/HbO_2,max)100$

| 98.7 | 98.2 | 97.4 | 96.9 | 95.9 | 94.1 | 90.9 | 85.1 | 74.7 | 57.5 | 32.4 | 9.6 |
|---|---|---|---|---|---|---|---|---|---|---|---|

$PO_2$ (mm Hg): 10 20 30 40 50 60 70 80 90 100 120 140

**FIG. 7.** A worksheet showing a difference in $PO_2$ between alveolar gas and mixed pulmonary capillary blood produced by a roughly normal spectrum of $\dot{V}_A/\dot{Q}$ distributions. These data, showing a $\Delta PO_2$ of 5 mm Hg, serve as the starting point for the data processing performed in a similar worksheet in Fig. 8. The data tabulated at the bottom of the figure (rows A, B, C, D) represent the "standard" Hb-$O_2$ dissociation curve: In normal man with HbA, pH = 7.4, temperature = 37°C, and [Hb] = 147 g/liter. (Data of J. W. Severinghaus, *J. Appl. Physiol.*, 46:599, 1979.)

difference between the $P_{O_2}$ of the mixed alveolar gas (102 mm Hg) and the $P_{O_2}$ of the mixed pulmonary venous blood (97 mm Hg). $P\bar{p}\bar{v}_{O_2}$ is 5 mm Hg less than $P_{A_{O_2}}$, simply because of a relatively normal distribution of $\dot{V}_A/\dot{Q}$ ratios in this model lung. Were the mismatching to get worse, as occurs during diseases which distort pulmonary architecture and function, the difference could get far larger and might lead to tissue hypoxia, even at rest.

## PHYSIOLOGICAL R-L SHUNT

In the introductory respiration chapter we briefly discussed two factors that tended to cause arterial $P_{O_2}$ ($Pa_{O_2}$) to be less than alveolar $P_{O_2}$ ($P_{A_{O_2}}$), even in normal, healthy people. We have just discussed one of them in more detail, showing that a reasonably normal spectrum of $\dot{V}_A/\dot{Q}$ ratios can cause blood $P_{O_2}$ to be less than $P_{A_{O_2}}$, even though there was equilibrium for $P_{O_2}$ between blood and gas in each alveolus. The other factor to be considered is the existence of a small R-L shunt in normal, healthy people. The term, "right-to-left shunt" describes a situation in which venous blood (deoxygenated, low $P_{O_2}$) mixes with arterial blood without having been arterialized in the lungs. Said another way, venous blood normally returns to the right side of the heart to be sent to the lungs, and only then is fed into the left side of the heart to be pumped into the systemic arteries. An R-L shunt occurs when some of this "right-sided blood" shunts to the left side *without* having been arterialized in the lungs.

In normal, healthy people about 2% of the cardiac output is involved in this normal, physiological R-L shunt. The anatomical basis of the shunt is probably twofold. First, some of the bronchial circulation (systemic arterial circulation which perfuses the airways of the lungs) returns to the left heart via the pulmonary veins. Secondly, although much of the coronary circulation returns to the right atrium through the coronary sinus, some of the coronary venous blood returns directly to the chamber of the left ventricle via the thebesian veins. Let us examine the effect of this venous admixture by imposing a 2% R-L shunt upon blood which has been exposed to the $\dot{V}_A/\dot{Q}$ mismatching just discussed. The 5 liters of blood which went through our three-compartment lung model carried a total of 973.5 ml $O_2$ toward the left heart per minute, giving each liter a content of 194.7 ml $O_2$. Figure 8 shows the effect of allowing a venous admixture of 2% into this 5 liters of blood. Category 1 shows that the $P_{A_{O_2}}$ is still 102 mm Hg. Categories 5, 6, and 7 of compartment I describe the characteristics of the blood which has been exposed to the $\dot{V}_A/\dot{Q}$ mismatch but has not had the R-L shunt added yet. Categories 5, 6, and 7 of compartment II show that we are now adding mixed venous blood ($O_2$ content = 148 ml/liter) at a rate of flow which is 2% of the total ($0.02 \times 5 = 0.1$), which will carry 14.8 ml $O_2$/min toward the left heart. Thus, the total amount of $O_2$ carried is 988.3 ml/min. It is carried by a total of 5.1 liters blood/min, for a final mixed content of 193.8 ml $O_2$/liter. Looking along row A of the tabular data shows that this content corresponds to a $P_{O_2}$ of about 89 mm Hg.

## CATEGORIES

| | 1 | 2 | 3 | 4 | 5 | 6 | 7 | 8 | 9 | 10 | 11 | 12 |
|---|---|---|---|---|---|---|---|---|---|---|---|---|
| C O M P A R T M E N T | $P_AO_2$ | $\dot{V}_A$ | $[O_2]$ as $[HbO_2]$ | $[O_2]$diss. | $(3)+(4)$ | $\dot{Q}$ | $(5)\times(6)$ | Total $O_2$ Carried By Blood | Mixed Blood % Sat. | Mixed Blood $PO_2$ | Gas – Bl $\Delta PO_2$ | Overall $\dot{V}_A/\dot{Q}$ |
| | mm Hg | liter/min | ml/liter | ml/liter | ml/liter | liter/min | ml $O_2$/min | $[O_2]$ of Mixed Blood (ml/liter) | | (mm Hg) | (mm Hg) | |
| I | | | | | 194.7 | 5.0 | 973.5 | | | | | |
| II | | | | | 148 | 0.1 | 14.8 | | | | | |
| III | | | | | | | | | | | | |
| IV | | | | | | | | | | | | |
| TOTALS, MEANS, MIXED GAS, BL | Mean $P_AO_2$ 102 | Total $\dot{V}_A$ | | | | Total $\dot{Q}$ 5.1 | 988.3 | 193.8 | 96 | 89 | 13 | 0.8 |

### $PO_2$ (mm Hg)

10  20  30  40  50  60  70  80  90  100  120  140

| | 10 | 20 | 30 | 40 | 50 | 60 | 70 | 80 | 90 | 100 | 120 | 140 |
|---|---|---|---|---|---|---|---|---|---|---|---|---|
| **A** WHOLE BLOOD $[O_2]$ ml $O_2$/liter blood | 19.2 | 64.4 | 114 | 148 | 169 | 181 | 187 | 191 | 194 | 195 | 197 | 199 |
| **B** DISSOLVED $[O_2]$ ml $O_2$/liter blood | 0.3 | 0.6 | 0.9 | 1.2 | 1.5 | 1.8 | 2.1 | 2.4 | 2.7 | 3.0 | 3.6 | 4.2 |
| **C** $[O_2]$ combined with Hb ml $O_2$/liter blood | 18.9 | 63.8 | 113 | 147 | 168 | 179 | 185 | 189 | 191 | 192 | 193 | 194 |
| **D** % Saturation of Hb ($HbO_2/HbO_{2,max}$)100 | 9.6 | 32.4 | 57.5 | 74.7 | 85.1 | 90.9 | 94.1 | 95.9 | 96.9 | 97.4 | 98.2 | 98.7 |

**FIG. 8.** A worksheet showing an alveolar to arterial $\Delta PO_2$ produced by superimposing a 2% R-L shunt on a roughly normal spectrum of $\dot{V}_A/\dot{Q}$ distributions. To 5 liters/min of blood whose composition was determined by the $\dot{V}_A/\dot{Q}$ distribution in Fig. 7 is added 0.1 liters/min of mixed venous blood via a R-L shunt. The result is a $Pa_{O_2}$ 13 mm Hg less than the $PA_{O_2}$. The tabulated data at the bottom of the figure (rows, A, B, C, D) represent the "standard" Hb-$O_2$ dissociation curve: In normal man with HbA, pH = 7.4, temperature = 37°C, and [Hb] = 147 g/liter. (Data of J. W. Severinghaus, *J. Appl. Physiol.*, 46:599, 1979.)

Thus, the alveolar $P_{O_2}$ is 102 mm Hg; blood which has been exposed to a roughly normal spectrum of $\dot{V}_A/\dot{Q}$ mismatching has a $P_{O_2}$ of only 97, 5 mm Hg less; and blood which has been subjected both to the $\dot{V}_A/\dot{Q}$ mismatching and the normal 2% R-L shunt has a $P_{O_2}$ of only 89 mm Hg. This last blood, which is now arterial blood, thus has a $P_{O_2}$ which is 13 mm Hg less than that of the alveolar gas. This is a not unreasonable difference between alveolar and arterial $P_{O_2}$ in normal persons, breathing air at sea level, and arterial $P_{O_2}$ of about 90 mm Hg under these conditions is quite commonly found.

## PATHOLOGY AND DIFFERENTIAL DIAGNOSIS—A BRIEF WORD

Any and all of these processes (gas diffusion between alveolar gas and blood, $\dot{V}_A/\dot{Q}$ mismatching, R-L shunting) can become far worse in pathological situations and cause arterial hypoxemia. Clearly, a detailed coverage of pulmonary function tests as used in the diagnosis of pathology is far beyond the scope of this text. Nevertheless, the author feels that a brief statement about the differential diagnosis among these three potential causes of arterial hypoxemia may underscore the relevance of the material in this chapter.

First, it should be said that rarely, if ever, does pathology cause hypoxemia through a worsening of only one of these processes. In pulmonary emphysema, for example, the $\Delta P_{O_2}$ at each of the three points in the $O_2$ cascade will likely be greater than normal. The diffusion path may be increased in length while the surface area may be decreased, leading to nonequilibrium for $P_{O_2}$ between each alveolus and its pulmonary capillary blood, thus contributing to a larger than normal difference between $P_{A_{O_2}}$ and $Pa_{O_2}$. The $\dot{V}_A/\dot{Q}$ mismatching may be worse than usual, thereby contributing more than usual to a difference between $P_{A_{O_2}}$ and $Pa_{O_2}$. Finally, there may be a population of alveoli that are totally nonventilated, their perfusion thereby becoming an R-L shunt ($\dot{V}_A/\dot{Q}$ ratio = 0); or, there may be an abnormal extrapulmonary R-L shunt occurring via an atrail or ventricular septal defect, or patent ductus arteriosus. In either of these situations, the R-L shunt world contribute an abnormally large increment to a difference between $P_{A_{O_2}}$ and $Pa_{O_2}$.

It is possible to conduct a simple test in a hypoxemic patient which may confirm the existence of a large R-L shunt. One simply raises the $F_{I_{O_2}}$ to 0.5 or more while monitoring the arterial Hb saturation. Nonsaturation under these circumstances proves the existence of a large R-L shunt; saturation gives very little additional information. The reasoning is as follows: Suppose the hypoxemia and desaturation is primarily due to impaired diffusion causing nonequilibrium between alveolar gas and pulmonary capillary blood. The mean diffusion gradient for $P_{O_2}$ is simply not large enough with this diffusion difficulty to raise $Ppc_{O_2}$ near 100 mm Hg, which is approximately what $P_{A_{O_2}}$ will be. By increasing $F_{I_{O_2}}$, however, we may raise $P_{A_{O_2}}$ to 400 mm Hg or more. Since the $P_{O_2}$ of the mixed venous blood will not change more than a few millimeters of mercury under these circumstances, the $P_{O_2}$ driving $O_2$ from alveolar gas to pulmonary capillary blood will be increased some sevenfold. Even though there is still no equilibrium between the $PA_{O_2}$ and $Ppc_{O_2}$, the latter will now be raised well above 100 mm Hg, resulting in saturation of Hb. Suppose the hypoxemia and desaturation is primarily due to worsened $\dot{V}A/\dot{Q}$ mismatching, but there are no alveoli in which the ratio is zero (no intrapulmonary R-L shunts). When we raise $FI_{O_2}$ greatly, any alveoli, no matter how poorly ventilated, will still have their $PO_2$ raised above 100 mm Hg. Thus, in this hypothetical case as well, there will be saturation of Hb with $O_2$. Finally, suppose that the hypoxemia and desaturation is primarily due to a large (greater than 20% of cardiac output) R-L shunt. The high $FI_{O_2}$ will result in a greatly decreased $PA_{O_2}$, which will load some additional $O_2$ onto the blood perfusing the "good" alveoli (not much extra, however, since the Hb is already saturated 97.5% at a $PO_2$ of 100 mm Hg). There is some extra $O_2$ which is dissolved at this greater $PO_2$, (but, again, not much). The blood going through the large R-L shunt, however, has very much less $O_2$ than does the arterialized blood. Thus, the slight extra amount of $O_2$ on the arterialized blood doesn't begin to compensate for the much reduced $O_2$ content of the shunted blood. The arterial blood therefore remains desaturated, confirming the existence of a large R-L shunt. (Quantitative examples of this calculation are included in problems 3 and 4 at the end of this chapter.)

## REFERENCES

1. Comroe, J. H., Jr. (1974): *Physiology of Respiration.* Year Book Medical Publishers, Chicago.
2. West, J. B. (1974): *Resiratory Physiology: The Essentials.* Williams & Wilkins, Baltimore.
3. West, J. B. (1977): *Ventilation/Blood Flow and Gas Exchange.* Blackwell, Oxford.

## PROBLEMS

1. The primary defect in a patient is a thickened membrane between alveolar gas and pulmonary capillary blood. He is at rest and breathing air in the steady state. Which of the combinations of gas pressures (a-e) is most consistent with that condition?

|    | $PA_{CO_2}$ (mm Hg) | $PA_{O_2}$ (mm Hg) | $Pa_{CO_2}$ (mm Hg) | $Pa_{O_2}$ (mm Hg) |
|----|----|----|----|----|
| a. | 30 | 114 | 32 | 50 |
| b. | 40 | 104 | 40 | 45 |
| c. | 40 | 104 | 40 | 94 |
| d. | 40 | 104 | 60 | 104 |
| e. | 40 | 104 | 60 | 84 |

2. Use the three-compartment model of the lung (shown in Fig. 9) to answer questions A and B. You may also find the worksheet in Fig. 10 to be useful.

   A. The mean alveolar $PO_2$ in mm Hg is closest to
      a. 120
      b. 100

| Compart-ments | $\dot{V}_A$ | $\dot{Q}$ | $\dot{V}_A/\dot{Q}$ | $P_{A_{O_2}}$ |
|---|---|---|---|---|
| I | 0.75 | 0.5 | 1.5 | 120 |
| II | 1.2 | 1.0 | 1.2 | 100 |
| III | 2.0 | 3.5 | 0.57 | 80 |

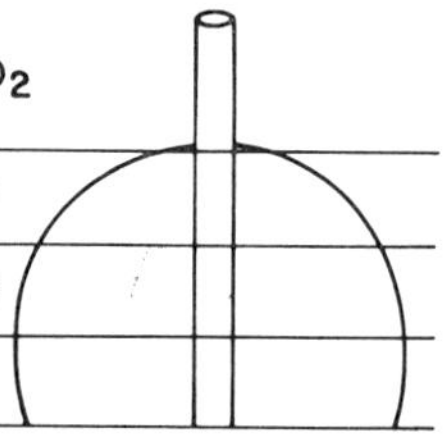

**FIG. 9.** A three-compartment model of the lung providing some of the data for problem 2A and B.

    c. 94
    d. 88
    e. 80

B. The difference in $P_{O_2}$ between mixed alveolar gas and mixed pulmonary venous blood is closest to
    a. 5 mm Hg
    b. 9 mm Hg
    c. 14 mm Hg
    d. 19 mm Hg
    e. 24 mm Hg

3. The following measurements were obtained in a patient with a normal Hb concentration and an oxygen consumption of 300 ml $O_2$/min, STPD.

|  | $O_2$ Content (ml/liter blood) | Mean pressure (mm Hg) |
|---|---|---|
| Radial artery | 175.0 | 85 |
| Right atrium | 135.0 | 7 |
| Pulmonary artery | 135.0 | 95 |
| Left atrium | Saturated | 20 |

A. The flow through the shunt is closest to
    a. 1.9 liters/min
    b. 2.5 liters/min
    c. 2.9 liters/min
    d. 4.6 liters/min
    e. 7.5 liters/min

B. The pulmonary vascular resistance is closest to
    a.  4 mm Hg/(liter/min)
    b.  8 mm Hg/(liter/min)

CATEGORIES

| | 1 | 2 | 3 | 4 | 5 | 6 | 7 | 8 | 9 | 10 | 11 | 12 |
|---|---|---|---|---|---|---|---|---|---|---|---|---|
| COMPARTMENT | $P_AO_2$ mm Hg | $\dot{V}_A$ liter/min | $[O_2]$ as $[HbO_2]$ ml/liter | $[O_2]$diss. ml/liter | (3) + (4) ml/liter | $\dot{Q}$ liter/min | (5) × (6) ml $O_2$/min | Total $O_2$ Carried By Blood | Mixed Blood % Sat. | Mixed Blood $PO_2$ (mm Hg) | Gas – Bl $\Delta PO_2$ (mm Hg) | $\dot{V}_A/\dot{Q}$ |
| I | | | | | | Total $\dot{Q}$ | Total $O_2$ Carried By Blood | $[O_2]$ of Mixed Blood (ml/liter) | | | | |
| II | | | | | | | | | | | | |
| III | | | | | | | | | | | | |
| IV | | | | | | | | | | | | |
| TOTALS, MEANS, MIXED GAS, BL | Mean $P_AO_2$ | Total $\dot{V}_A$ | | | | | | | | | Overall $\dot{V}_A/\dot{Q}$ | |

$PO_2$ (mm Hg)

10  20  30  40  50  60  70  80  90 100 120 140

| | | | | | | | | | | | | |
|---|---|---|---|---|---|---|---|---|---|---|---|---|
| A WHOLE BLOOD [O2] ml O2/liter blood | 19.2 | 64.4 | 114 | 148 | 169 | 181 | 187 | 191 | 194 | 195 | 197 | 199 |
| B DISSOLVED [O2] ml O2/liter blood | 0.3 | 0.6 | 0.9 | 1.2 | 1.5 | 1.8 | 2.1 | 2.4 | 2.7 | 3.0 | 3.6 | 4.2 |
| C [O2] combined with Hb ml O2/liter blood | 18.9 | 63.8 | 113 | 147 | 168 | 179 | 185 | 189 | 191 | 192 | 193 | 194 |
| D % Saturation of Hb (HbO2/HbO2,max)100 | 9.6 | 32.4 | 57.5 | 74.7 | 85.1 | 90.9 | 94.1 | 95.9 | 96.9 | 97.4 | 98.2 | 98.7 |

**FIG. 10.** Worksheet to be used in solving problem 2A and B. The bottom of this figure (rows A, B, C, D) represents the "standard" Hb-$O_2$ dissociation curve in tabular form: In normal man with HbA, pH = 7.4, temperature = 37°C, and [Hb] = 147 g/liter. (Data of J. W. Severinghaus, *J. Appl. Physiol.*, 46:599, 1979.)

    c. 12 mm Hg/(liter/min)
    d. 16 mm Hg/(liter/min)
    e. 20 mm Hg/(liter/min)

C. These data most likely represent
    a. a shunt from right atrium to left atrium
    b. a shunt from left atrium to right atrium
    c. a shunt from right ventricle to left ventricle
    d. a hunt from left ventricle to right ventricle
    e. an arterio venous fistula in the left leg

4. Using both the model in Fig. 11 of a large R-L shunt and the worksheet
in Fig. 12, calculate $Pa_{O_2}$ and the percent saturation of arterial blood with
$O_2$ when:

A. breathing room air
B. breathing 100% $O_2$

## ANSWERS

1. If the primary defect here is thickened membranes between alveolar gas
and pulmonary capillary blood, there ought to be a considerable increase

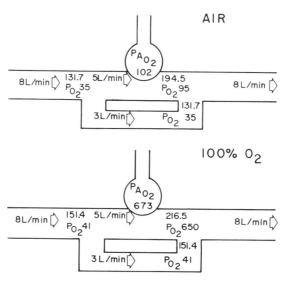

**FIG. 11.** A model of lung with a large R-L shunt. The top of the figure depicts values while breathing air, and the bottom depicts those values while breathing 100% $O_2$. The numbers in brackets are the $O_2$ contents of whole blood in ml/liter blood. These data, together with the worksheet shown in Fig. 12 are to be used in solving problem 4A and B.

# CATEGORIES

| | 1 | 2 | 3 | 4 | 5 | 6 | 7 | 8 | 9 | 10 | 11 | 12 |
|---|---|---|---|---|---|---|---|---|---|---|---|---|
| COMPARTMENT | $P_AO_2$ mm Hg | $\dot{V}_A$ liter/min | $[O_2]$ as $[HbO_2]$ ml/liter | $[O_2]$diss. ml/liter | $(3)+(4)$ ml/liter | $\dot{Q}$ liter/min | $(5)\times(6)$ ml $O_2$/min | Total $O_2$ Carried By Blood | Mixed Blood % Sat. | Mixed Blood $PO_2$ (mm Hg) | Gas – Bl $\Delta PO_2$ (mm Hg) | Overall $\dot{V}_A/\dot{Q}$ |
| I | | | | | | | | | | | | |
| II | | | | | | | | | | | | |
| III | | | | | | | | | | | | |
| IV | | | | | | | | | | | | |
| TOTALS, MEANS, MIXED GAS, BL | Mean $P_AO_2$ | Total $\dot{V}_A$ | | | | Total $\dot{Q}$ | | $[O_2]$ of Mixed Blood (ml/liter) | | | | |

## $PO_2$ (mm Hg)

| | 10 | 20 | 30 | 40 | 50 | 60 | 70 | 80 | 90 | 100 | 120 | 140 |
|---|---|---|---|---|---|---|---|---|---|---|---|---|
| A — WHOLE BLOOD $[O_2]$ ml $O_2$/liter blood | 19.2 | 64.4 | 114 | 148 | 169 | 181 | 187 | 191 | 194 | 195 | 197 | 199 |
| B — DISSOLVED $[O_2]$ ml $O_2$/liter blood | 0.3 | 0.6 | 0.9 | 1.2 | 1.5 | 1.8 | 2.1 | 2.4 | 2.7 | 3.0 | 3.6 | 4.2 |
| C — $[O_2]$ combined with Hb ml $O_2$/liter blood | 18.9 | 63.8 | 113 | 147 | 168 | 179 | 185 | 189 | 191 | 192 | 193 | 194 |
| D — % Saturation of Hb $(HbO_2/HbO_{2,max})100$ | 9.6 | 32.4 | 57.5 | 74.7 | 85.1 | 90.9 | 94.1 | 95.9 | 96.9 | 97.4 | 98.2 | 98.7 |

**FIG. 12.** Worksheet to be used in solving problem 4A and B. The bottom of this figure (rows A, B, C, D) represents the "standard" $HbO_2$ dissociation curve in tabular form. Normal man, HbA, pH = 7.4, Temp = 37°C, [Hb] = 147 g/liter. (Data of J. W. Severinghaus, *J. Appl. Physiol.*, 46:599, 1979.)

## CATEGORIES

| | 1 | 2 | 3 | 4 | 5 | 6 | 7 | 8 | 9 | 10 | 11 | 12 |
|---|---|---|---|---|---|---|---|---|---|---|---|---|
| C O M P A R T M E N T | $P_AO_2$ mm Hg | $\dot{V}_A$ liter/min | $[O_2]$ as $[HbO_2]$ ml/liter | $[O_2]$diss. ml/liter | (3) + (4) ml/liter | $\dot{Q}$ liter/min | (5) × (6) ml $O_2$/min | Total $[O_2]$ of Mixed Blood (ml/liter) | Mixed Blood % Sat. | Mixed Blood $PO_2$ (mm Hg) | Gas − Bl $\Delta PO_2$ (mm Hg) | $\dot{V}_A/\dot{Q}$ |
| I | 120 | 0.75 | 193 | 3.6 | 197 | 0.5 | 98.5 | | | | | 1.5 |
| II | 100 | 1.25 | 192 | 3.0 | 195 | 1.0 | 195 | | | | | 1.25 |
| III | 80 | 2.0 | 189 | 2.4 | 191 | 3.5 | 668.5 | | | | | 0.57 |
| IV | | | | | | | | | | | | |
| TOTALS, MEANS, MIXED GAS, BL | Mean $P_AO_2$ 93.8 | Total $\dot{V}_A$ 4.0 | | | | Total $\dot{Q}$ 5.0 | 962 | 192.4 | 96.4 | 85 | Overall $\dot{V}_A/\dot{Q}$ 9 | 0.8 |

### $PO_2$ (mm Hg)

| | 10 | 20 | 30 | 40 | 50 | 60 | 70 | 80 | 90 | 100 | 120 | 140 |
|---|---|---|---|---|---|---|---|---|---|---|---|---|
| A WHOLE BLOOD $[O_2]$ ml $O_2$/liter blood | 19.2 | 64.4 | 114 | 148 | 169 | 181 | 187 | 191 | 194 | 195 | 197 | 199 |
| B DISSOLVED $[O_2]$ ml $O_2$/liter blood | 0.3 | 0.6 | 0.9 | 1.2 | 1.5 | 1.8 | 2.1 | 2.4 | 2.7 | 3.0 | 3.6 | 4.2 |
| C $[O_2]$ combined with Hb ml $O_2$/liter blood | 18.9 | 63.8 | 113 | 147 | 168 | 179 | 185 | 189 | 191 | 192 | 193 | 194 |
| D % Saturation of Hb $(HbO_2/HbO_{2,max})100$ | 9.6 | 32.4 | 57.5 | 74.7 | 85.1 | 90.9 | 94.1 | 95.9 | 96.9 | 97.4 | 98.2 | 98.7 |

**FIG. 13.** Worksheet showing answers to problem 2A and B. "Standard" $HbO_2$ dissociation curve in tabular form. Normal man, HbA, pH = 7.4, Temp = 37°C, [Hb] = 147 g/liter. (Data of J. W. Severinghaus: *J. Appl. Physiol.* 46:599, 1979.)

in the usual difference in $P_{O_2}$ between those two compartments. By this criterion, (a), (b), and (e) are possible answers. However, (e) can be ruled out immediately because there's no way that the defect could result in an arterial $P_{CO_2}$ that is 20 mm Hg above the alveolar. Alternatives (a) and (b) have arterial $P_{O_2}$ values that are low enough to be in the strongly stimulatory range for the peripheral chemoreceptors; however, only (a) shows evidence of the hyperventilation that should occur ($P_{A_{CO_2}}$ and $P_{a_{CO_2}}$ being about three-fourths that of a normal, sea-level male). Neither (a) nor (b) show a significant difference between the partial pressures of $CO_2$ in alveolar gas and arterial blood, because $CO_2$ is some 20 times as diffusible as is $O_2$. Alternative (a) is correct.

2. See Fig. 13. The reasonably normal distribution of $\dot{V}_A/\dot{Q}$ ratios has resulted in a difference of 9 mm Hg between alveolar and mixed pulmonary capillary $P_{O_2}$.

3. I usually find it helpful to diagram problems such as this, put in my numbers as I calculate them, and thereby visualize the situation more easily (see Fig. 14). The $\dot{V}_{O_2}$ of 300 ml/min together with the $O_2$ contents of 175 and 135 ml $O_2$/liter in the arteries and right atrium, respectively, enable one to use the Fick principle to calculate systemic $\dot{Q}$ to be 7.5 liters/min. The $\dot{V}_{O_2}$ at the lungs must also be 300 ml/min, and pulmonary artery $O_2$ content is

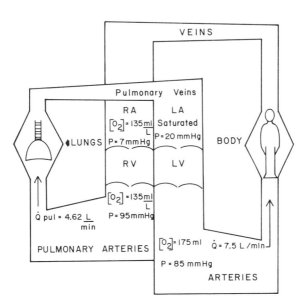

**FIG. 14.** A model of the cardiovascular and respiratory systems to serve as an aid in the solution of problem 3A–C.

## CATEGORIES

| | 1 $P_AO_2$ mm Hg | 2 $\dot{V}_A$ liter/min | 3 [O₂] as [HbO₂] ml/liter | 4 [O₂]diss. ml/liter | 5 (3)+(4) ml/liter | 6 $\dot{Q}$ liter/min | 7 (5) × (6) ml O₂/min | 8 Total O₂ Carried By Blood — [O₂] of Mixed Blood (ml/liter) | 9 Mixed Blood % Sat. | 10 Mixed Blood $PO_2$ (mm Hg) | 11 Gas − Bl $\Delta PO_2$ (mm Hg) | 12 $\dot{V}_A/\dot{Q}$ |
|---|---|---|---|---|---|---|---|---|---|---|---|---|
| I | | | | | 194.5 | 5 | 972.5 | | | | | |
| II | | | | | 131.7 | 3 | 395.1 | | | | | |
| III | | | | | | | | | | | | |
| IV | | | | | | | | | | | | |
| TOTALS, MEANS, MIXED GAS, BL | Mean $P_AO_2$ 102 | Total $\dot{V}_A$ 4.0 | | | | Total $\dot{Q}$ 8.0 | 1367.6 | 171.0 | 86 | 52 | 50 | Overall $\dot{V}_A/\dot{Q}$ |

## $PO_2$ (mm Hg)

| | 10 | 20 | 30 | 40 | 50 | 60 | 70 | 80 | 90 | 100 | 120 | 140 |
|---|---|---|---|---|---|---|---|---|---|---|---|---|
| **A** WHOLE BLOOD [O₂] ml O₂/liter blood | 19.2 | 64.4 | 114 | 148 | 169 | 181 | 187 | 191 | 194 | 195 | 197 | 199 |
| **B** DISSOLVED [O₂] ml O₂/liter blood | 0.3 | 0.6 | 0.9 | 1.2 | 1.5 | 1.8 | 2.1 | 2.4 | 2.7 | 3.0 | 3.6 | 4.2 |
| **C** [O₂] combined with Hb ml O₂/liter blood | 18.9 | 63.8 | 113 | 147 | 168 | 179 | 185 | 189 | 191 | 192 | 193 | 194 |
| **D** % Saturation of Hb (HbO₂/HbO₂,max)100 | 9.6 | 32.4 | 57.5 | 74.7 | 85.1 | 90.9 | 94.1 | 95.9 | 96.9 | 97.4 | 98.2 | 98.7 |

**FIG. 15.** Worksheet showing answer to problem 4A. "Standard" HbO₂ dissociation curve in tabular form. Normal man, HbA, pH = 7.4, Temp = 37°C, [Hb] = 147 g/liter. (Data of J. W. Severinghaus: *J. Appl. Physiol.* 46:599, 1979.)

CATEGORIES

| | 1 | 2 | 3 | 4 | 5 | 6 | 7 | 8 | 9 | 10 | 11 | 12 |
|---|---|---|---|---|---|---|---|---|---|---|---|---|
| C O M P A R T M E N T | $P_AO_2$ mm Hg | $\dot{V}_A$ liter/min | $[O_2]$ as $[HbO_2]$ ml/liter | $[O_2]$diss. ml/liter | (3) + (4) ml/liter | $\dot{Q}$ liter/min | (5) × (6) ml $O_2$/min | Total $O_2$ Carried By Blood | | | | $\dot{V}_A/\dot{Q}$ |
| I | | | | | 216.5 | 5.0 | 1082.4 | | | | | |
| II | | | | | 151.4 | 3.0 | 454.1 | | | | | |
| III | | | | | | | | | | | | |
| IV | | | | | | | | | | | | |
| TOTALS, MEANS, MIXED GAS, BL | Mean $P_AO_2$ 673 | Total $\dot{V}_A$ 4.0 | | | | Total $\dot{Q}$ 8.0 | 1536.5 | $[O_2]$ of Mixed Blood (ml/liter) 192.1 | Mixed Blood % Sat. 96.4 | Mixed Blood $PO_2$ (mm Hg) 85 | Gas - Bl $\Delta PO_2$ (mm Hg) 588 | Overall $\dot{V}_A/\dot{Q}$ |

## $PO_2$ (mm Hg)

10 20 30 40 50 60 70 80 90 100 120 140

| | | | | | | | | | | | | |
|---|---|---|---|---|---|---|---|---|---|---|---|---|
| A WHOLE BLOOD $[O_2]$ ml $O_2$/liter blood | 19.2 | 64.4 | 114 | 148 | 169 | 181 | 187 | 191 | 194 | 195 | 197 | 199 |
| B DISSOLVED $[O_2]$ ml $O_2$/liter blood | 0.3 | 0.6 | 0.9 | 1.2 | 1.5 | 1.8 | 2.1 | 2.4 | 2.7 | 3.0 | 3.6 | 4.2 |
| C $[O_2]$ combined with Hb ml $O_2$/liter blood | 18.9 | 63.8 | 113 | 147 | 168 | 179 | 185 | 189 | 191 | 192 | 193 | 194 |
| D % Saturation of Hb $(HbO_2/HbO_{2,max})100$ | 9.6 | 32.4 | 57.5 | 74.7 | 85.1 | 90.9 | 94.1 | 95.9 | 96.9 | 97.4 | 98.2 | 98.7 |

**FIG. 16.** Worksheet showing answer to problem 4B. "Standard" $HbO_2$ dissociation curve in tabular form. Normal man, HbA, pH = 7.4, Temp = 37°C, [Hb] = 147 g/liter. (Data of J. W. Severinghaus: *J. Appl. Physiol.* 46:599, 1979.)

135 ml/liter but the left atrial $O_2$ content is described as "saturated." Since the patient has a normal Hb concentration, however, we know that his $O_2$ capacity must be about 200 ml $O_2$/liter. Using that we get a pulmonary $\dot{Q}$ of 4.62 liters/min, or 2.88 liters/min less than the systemic. Therefore there is a shunt of 2.88 liters/min, but where? It's not left-to-right in the heart since the $O_2$ content of right atrial and pulmonary arterial blood is the same. It *is* a R-L shunt, since left atrial $O_2$ content is 200 ml/liter while arterial content is only 175! The shunt can't be intraatrial since the left atrial blood is saturated, and since the pressure gradient is in the wrong direction! It could be intraventricular or through a patent ductus arteriosus; the pressures on the right side are abnormally high in the arteries, and by inference, in the ventricles. So, answer to both **A** and **C** is (c). **B** is a straightforward application of Ohm's law $R = \Delta P/\dot{Q} = (95 - 20)$ mm Hg/(4.62 liter/min), or about 16 mm Hg/(liter/min), which is alternative (d).

4. **A:** See Fig. 15. **B:** See Fig. 16. Note that 100% $O_2$ does not lead to normal saturation of arterial blood in this case of a large R-L shunt.

# 8

---

# *Regulation of Breathing*

It was mentioned briefly in the first of the chapters on respiration that the muscles of the respiratory system, having no inherent pacemaker of their own, must be induced to contract rhythmically by some system of regulation in the brain. Such a system must be capable of generating impulses in the motor nerves to the muscles of breathing, which will result in exchanges between environment and alveolar gas of widely differing magnitudes, depending on the particular environment in which the organism finds itself, and on the particular activity in which it is engaged. Thus, while resting ventilation may be 5–7 liters/min, ventilation during long-term residence at 15,000 ft. may be 10 liters/min, and that during heavy exercise may be as high as 75–100 liters/min.

The central nervous system control of the cardiovascular system is essentially completely automatic, incapable of appreciable voluntary control, and housed in the brainstem. Respiration also has this automatic type of regulatory system housed in the brainstem. It responds to a whole variety of information about activity and environment from mechano- and chemoreceptors and reflexly adjusts breathing to best provide for the person's needs. It works completely without our conscious intervention during sleep, while under anesthesia, or while we're awake but not thinking about breathing.

But we use our respiratory muscles for so many activities besides breathing. These activities include speaking, singing, whistling, straining at stool, aiding in childbirth, coughing, sniffing, clearing our throats, blowing our noses, holding our breaths as we swim underwater, playing musical instruments, and many, many more. The voluntary activities among these are under the control of the cerebral cortex, and the neural pathways between cortex and respiratory muscle motoneurons are separate from those emanating from the brainstem control system. There must be interaction between these two control systems, however. We can easily override the automatic system for a time voluntarily, as we do when breath-holding. Here, the cerebrum is suppressing the brainstem. Breath-holding can only proceed until the breaking point, however, at which point we must breathe regardless of motivation to the contrary. Thus, the automatic system can override the voluntary one. Of course, a more delicate and carefully coordinated interaction occurs during speech, singing, playing the tuba, etc.

The rest of the chapter will concentrate on the automatic control of breathing because it is that which is concerned with the maintenance of homeostasis of $P_{O_2}$, $P_{CO_2}$, and acid–base balance. First, there will be a discussion of what is known about the organization of respiratory neurons in the brainstem, the classic, poorly defined "respiratory centers" having given way to more specific localization of structures with functions. Next, the functioning of some pulmonary receptors will be discussed. The last part of the chapter will deal with chemical regulation of breathing, considering the peripheral chemoreceptors, the medullary chemoreceptors, and their interactions, in that order.

## NEURONS IN THE BRAINSTEM

Although it had been known since Galen's time that transection of the upper cervical spinal cord stopped breathing, our systematic knowledge of the organization of the respiratory neurons may have been furthered when a French physician introduced the guillotine in 1789. Curious observers must have noticed that respiratory movements persisted for a time in the head if the cut had been made below the brainstem.

Many studies aimed at refining this information followed, culminating in the classic studies of Lumsden in the early 1920's. By means of considerably more careful brainstem transections than those described above, he concluded that the central automatic respiratory system could be composed of four centers: Pneumotaxic, Apneustic, Expiratory, and Gasping Centers. His transections and the types of respiration that resulted are shown in Fig. 1. Transections made at level A (above the upper pons) caused no change in the respiration of an anesthetized animal. Cutting the vagi with or without this transection caused a slowing and deepening of respiration. A transection made in the mid-pons, just above the cerebral peduncles but below the Nucleus Parabrachialis (at level B) caused some slowing and deepening of respiration with the vagi left intact. When the vagi were cut, the transection at level B caused a series of prolonged inspirations, punctuated by very brief expirations. Lumsden termed this last respiratory pattern, "Apneustic Respiration," and believed that it was due to the activity of a tonically active center located in the lower pons which he called the Apneustic Center. Since the apneustic pattern had been unmasked by vagal and upper pontine section, he concluded that the apneustic center's activity normally was periodically inhibited (a) by impulses traveling in the vagus, and (b) by impulses from a center in the upper pons which he called the Pneumotaxic Center. When Lumsden transected at level C, removing the influence of the pons completely, he found regular respiratory rhythm to cease, being replaced either by a gasping pattern or by one dominated by expiratory spasms. These patterns did not seem to be consistently affected by vagal section. Thus were the gasping and expiratory centers postulated.

While few if any of these constructs are accepted today, the model has been

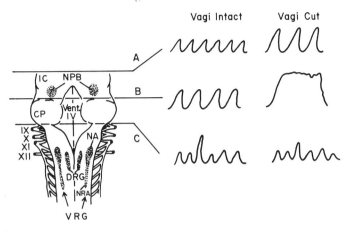

**FIG. 1.** Patterns of respiration after transection of the brainstem with vagi intact and transected. Transection above the nucleus parabrachialis has little effect on the pattern of involuntary breathing. Transection through or below the dorsal respiratory group and ventral respiratory group causes apnea. DRG, dorsal respiratory group; VRG, ventral respiratory group; IC, inferior colliculus; CP, cerebral peduncle; NA, nucleus ambiguus; NRA, nucleus retroambigualis; NPB, nucleus parabrachialis (pneumotaxic center). (Reproduced with permission from Mitchell, R. A. and A. J. Berger. Neural control of respiration. *Am. Rev. Respir. Dis.,* 111:206, 1975.)

involved in much of the research into the organization of respiratory neurons in the brain. The techniques used have included ablation, destruction, stimulation, neural recording, and histological marking; the task of working out the "wiring diagram" of the respiratory neurons has really only just begun. What follows is a brief description of our present understanding of the respiratory centers in the brainstem.

## PNEUMOTAXIC CENTER

The existence of the pneumotaxic center has been confirmed by many investigators. The neurons of which it is composed make up the nucleus parabrachialis in the dorsolateral rostral pons, labeled NPB in Fig. 1. It is generally agreed that its function is to modulate the output of the medullary respiratory centers (not unlike Lumsden's postulated function), but whether it can generate a respiratory rhythm on its own remains to be answered along with many other specific questions.

## APNEUSTIC CENTER

Modern workers agree with the early ones that destruction of the pneumotaxic center or its separation from the more caudal brainstem structures results in apneustic respiration when combined with vagotomy. Berger et al. suggest that the apneustic center may be the site of the normal inspiratory cutoff switch, that the various inputs which can terminate an inspiration project to this center. When inputs from above and from the vagus nerves are excluded, apneusis results. The specific neurons that constitute the apneustic center are not yet known.

## MEDULLARY CENTERS

It is now generally accepted that the medulla, when separated from all rostral structures but still connected with the spinal cord, *is* capable of maintaining rhythmic respiration. Intensive research efforts have recently identified the location of the neurons involved in respiration and have made progress in working out what each type does and how they interact with one another. The darkness in this area still far "outshines" the light, however, and it is not the purpose of this book to dwell at length with the cutting edge of research into any field. What follows, then, is a brief description of what *is* known.

Two dense bilateral aggregations of respiratory neurons have been identified, as shown in Figs. 1 and 2. One of these, mostly inspiratory cells, is found in the ventrolateral portion of the nucleus of the tractus solitarius (NTS) and has been called the dorsal respiratory group (DRG). The other, containing both inspiratory and expiratory cells, is found in the nucleus ambiguus (NA) and the nucleus retroambigualis (NRA) and has been called the ventral respiratory group (VRG).

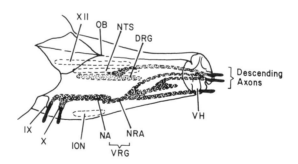

**FIG. 2.** Schematic representation of DRG and VRG with their efferent projections in the cat's brainstem. DRG located in the vicinity of NTS is the source of the rhythmic drive to contralateral phrenic motoneurons. VRG rostral division consists of cranial nerve motoneurons in NA which innervate the ipsilateral accessory muscles of respiration. The caudal division of VRG is the NRA and is the source of rhythmic drive to inspiratory and expiratory intercostal and probably abdominal expiratory motoneurons. These VRG respiratory neurons project contralaterally, but some inspiratory neurons project ipsilaterally. DRG, dorsal respiratory group; ION, inferior olivary nucleus; NA, nucleus ambiguus; NRA, nucleus retroambigualis; NTS, nucleus tractus solitarius; OB, obex; VH, ventral horn; VRG, ventral respiratory group; XII, hypoglossal nucleus. (Reproduced with permission from Mitchell, R. A. and Berger, A. J. Neural control of respiration. *Am. Rev. Respir. Dis.,* 111:206, 1975.)

## DRG

The cells in the DRG seem to be the "upper motor neurons" of many muscles of respiration, including the diaphragm. They also project to—and drive—the ventral respiratory group. These drives are rhythmic, but the site of rhythm generation does not seem to be within the DRG and is unlocated as of the writing of this chapter.

The DRG also seems to receive the afferents from some pulmonary and airway receptors. These include the Pulmonary Stretch Receptors (PSR), the Pulmonary Irritant Receptors (PIR), and receptors in the epipharynx and larynx.

## VRG

The cells of the VRG project to "distant" sites and drive either spinal respiratory motoneurons (intercostal and abdominal) or vagal motoneurons innervating the auxillary muscles of respiration. Again, the cells of the VRG are driven by the DRG; they are not responsible for the initial processing of sensory inputs.

## PULMONARY RECEPTORS

The receptors in the lung have been divided into the following three major classes: (a) PSR, (b) PIR, and (c) the Type J Receptors. The role of these receptors in normal regulation of breathing is poorly understood.

## PSR

These receptors are believed to lie in airway smooth muscle, to be activated by lung distension, to be slowly adapting, and to be innervated by large, myelinated vagal fibers. When activated by lung inflation, they cause a slowing of respiratory frequency due to a prolongation of expiratory time which is called the Hering-Breuer reflex, as well as bronchodilation, tachycardia, and vasoconstriction. The Hering-Breuer reflex is illustrated in Fig. 3 with data obtained from an anesthetized dog connected to a recording spirometer. Both records A and B show airway pressure ($P_{AW}$), esophageal pressure ($P_{ES}$), and change of lung volume as recorded from the spirometer. Record A shows four normal breaths followed by the clamping of the airway at the end of the fourth when the lung volume has just about returned to functional residual capacity (FRC). The animal attempts the next breath (as seen by the pressure changes in the airway and the esophagus) after an interval of time only slightly greater than normal. Record B shows two normal breaths in the same animal only minutes later, followed by clamping of the airway in the middle of the third breath, after inspiration and before expiration, at a lung volume of $FRC + V_T$. Because of the lung distension the animal does not attempt the next breath for about 20 seconds.

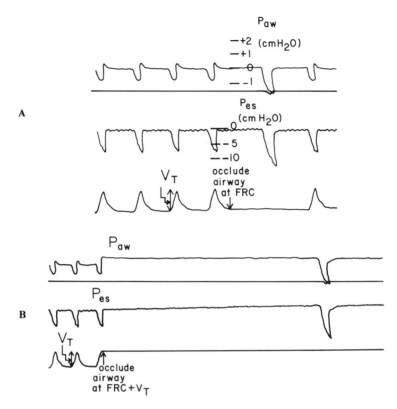

**FIG. 3. A:** The airway pressure (PAW), esophageal pressure (PES), and change in lung volume are recorded during several normal breaths and then while the tracheal cannula is clamped near FRC in an anesthetized dog. The next breath is attempted (see changes in PAW and PES) after a roughly normal interval of time. **B:** The same three parameters as in Fig. 3A are recorded during two normal breaths, and then during the clamping of the tracheal cannula at FRC + VI (at the peak of an inspiration). The next breath is attempted only after nine times the normal time interval, demonstrating the Hering-Breuer inflation reflex.

Obviously, the information from these receptors could be important in determining the rate and depth of breathing. To demonstrate their importance in the normal breath-to-breath adjustments of rate and depth, they must first be shown to cause reflexes in response to lung inflations in the normal range of breathing. In the dog and cat this test is easily passed. In man, however, the lung inflation must be 1.5–2 times the normal tidal volume in order to produce marked inhibition of breathing, thus raising questions about the role of the PSR in regulation of normal, resting breathing.

There is less doubt about their role in control of breathing during the inhalation of $CO_2$ (and, perhaps during exercise, with its greater fluctuation of $PCO_2$). Normally, inhaling $CO_2$ causes both frequency and tidal volume to increase.

Inhalation of $CO_2$ after the vagi are cut, however, causes increases in tidal volume only. The PSR could be the receptors involved here, since $Pco_2$ has been shown to decrease the PSR discharge of many animals. This would cause shorter expiratory phases, and thus could increase frequency. Lidocaine blockade of the vagus nerves in man has also been shown to alter the frequency–tidal volume relationship during $CO_2$ inhalation.

## PIR

These receptors are believed to lie between airway epithelial cells, to be activated by lung distension and some irritants, to be rapidly adapting, and to be innervated by myelinated vagal fibers. Their primary stimulus is probably the presence of chemical and/or particulate irritants, especially histamine, and the reflex effects of such stimulation include hyperpnea and bronchoconstriction.

There is controversy about the role of these receptors in control of breathing. The term "Irritant Receptors" was coined because investigators believed their primary stimulus to be the inhalation of chemical and/or particulate irritants. Some recent evidence indicates, however, that dog PIR are only occasionally excited by ammonia or cigarette smoke. It has been suggested that the PIR may be important in the reflex bronchoconstriction triggered by histamine release during an allergic asthmatic attack. Since the PIR seem also sensitive to changes in airway $Pco_2$, they may be involved in the rate:depth interaction during $CO_2$ inhalation.

### Type J or Juxtapulmonary Capillary Receptors

These receptors are believed to lie in the walls of the pulmonary capillaries and to be activated by an increase in pulmonary interstitial fluid such as might occur in pulmonary congestion and edema; they are rapidly adapting and are innervated by slowly conducting nonmyelinated vagal fibers. In the cat, they have also been shown to be activated by lung hyperinflation. The reflex effects caused by these receptors include apnea, hypotension, and bradycardia. There is little agreement at present about the role these receptors may play in the regulation of breathing.

## CHEMICAL CONTROL

The respiratory system cooperates with other systems of the body in maintaining homeostasis of $O_2$, $CO_2$, and $[H^+]$. The levels of these important substances are sensed by chemoreceptors which fall into two groups: the peripheral chemoreceptors and the central or medullary chemoreceptors. Changing the concentrations of $O_2$, $CO_2$, or $[H^+]$ causes reflex changes in breathing designed to minimize deviations from the normal "set point" of the substance in question. The peripheral and central chemoreceptors have very different structures, locations, and response characteristics from one another and are best considered separately before we get involved in their integrated responses to some physiologically important stimuli.

### Peripheral Chemoreceptors

The peripheral chemoreceptors themselves are divided into two groups, the carotid and aortic chemoreceptors. The carotid group is located in the carotid bodies, which are small nodules of tissue found bilaterally at the bifurcation of the common carotid arteries into the internal and external carotids. The aortic group is located in the aortic bodies, which are similar nodules of tissue found around the arch of the aorta and between the arch of the aorta and the pulmonary artery. Both groups are stimulated by decreased $Po_2$ in arterial blood and, to a lesser extent, by increased arterial $Pco_2$. The carotid group (but apparently not the aortic) is also stimulated by a decrease in arterial pH (without a concomitant rise in $Pco_2$). There is good evidence that the carotid chemoreceptors (and probably the aortic) can be stimulated also by a reduction in their normally enormous blood flows, such as might occur during a considerable fall in blood pressure, or during increased sympathetic activity.

While both groups of peripheral chemoreceptors are involved in cardiovascular as well as respiratory regulation, the carotid group exerts by far the dominant effects on respiration. In fact, investigators have reported over and over again that removal or denervation of the carotid chemoreceptors removes all measurable peripheral chemoreceptor effects on respiration. Thus, although the aortic chemoreceptors are important in cardiovascular regulation, we can confine our attentions to the response characteristics of the carotid chemoreceptors in a discussion of regulation of breathing.

### Carotid Chemoreceptors

The carotid bodies are responsible for the immediate increase in breathing which occurs when the arterial $Po_2$ is lowered; individuals without functional carotid bodies show no change in breathing, or even a depression of breathing, upon being made acutely hypoxic. Effective stimulation of the carotid bodies causes increases of ventilation very quickly (within a very few seconds).

Careful studies of the afferent information coming from carotid body chemoreceptors have pretty well characterized what information the brain receives from the carotid bodies in response to hypoxia, elevated $Pco_2$, and acidity. Figure 4 shows how the number of impulses/second in single afferent chemoreceptor fibers varies with $Pa_{O_2}$. The four different fibers were studied under conditions of normal $Pco_2$ in the same anesthetized cat, with great care being taken not to disturb the circulation and innervation of the carotid body. The records show the following: (a) There is small but nonzero activity even when $Pa_{O_2}$ is as high as 600 mm Hg. (b) This very low impulse activity increases little until

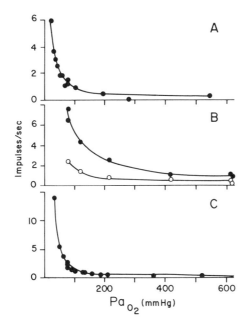

**FIG. 4.** The rate of chemoreceptor afferent discharges (impulses/second) in single fibers, plotted against the arterial $O_2$ tension (mm Hg), all from the same cat. **B** shows two fibers from the same strand; **A** and **C** are from single fibers. Arterial $Pco_2$ ranged between 28 and 34 mm Hg in all cases. Mean arterial blood pressure was 95 mm Hg in **A,** 97 mm Hg in **B,** and 123 mm Hg in **C.** (Reproduced with permission from Biscoe, T. J. et al., The frequency of nerve impulses in single carotid body chemoreceptor afferent fibers recorded *in vivo* with intact circulation. *J. Physiol. (Lond.),* 208:121, 1970.)

the $Pa_{O_2}$ is below the normal sea-level value of about 100 mm Hg. (c) From a $Pa_{O_2}$ of 100 mm Hg down to a $Pa_{O_2}$ in the low 30's, the number of impulses/ second increases more and more steeply, the curve tending asymptotically toward a maximum near 30 mm Hg.

All of these response characteristics are hard to explain mechanistically because we really don't understand how the carotid chemoreceptors work. Some of them are even hard to explain teleologically. For instance, what function can it serve to have the carotid bodies sending a small and roughly constant number of impulses to the central nervous system (CNS) between arterial $Po_2$ of 200 and 600 mm Hg? Why not zero?

It is easier to understand the function served by the impulse traffic's staying low until the $Pa_{O_2}$ goes below 100 mm Hg, and not really beginning to increase greatly until the $Pa_{O_2}$ has fallen to perhaps 50 mm Hg. The carotid chemoreceptors seem designed to guard against threats of diminished $O_2$ delivery to the tissues. As such, the insistence of the message they send to the CNS (which will determine the vigor of the ventilatory response) should depend on the desaturation of the arterial hemoglobin. At $Pa_{O_2}$ = 600 mm Hg, Hb will be about 99.8% saturated; it will still be 97.5% saturated when $Pa_{O_2}$ has fallen to 100 mm Hg. By the time $Pa_{O_2}$ has fallen to 50 mm Hg, however, the saturation will be about 85%, and it will be only about 75% at a $Pa_{O_2}$ of 40 mm Hg.

Figure 5 shows the familiar Hb dissociation curve of normal man together with (on the same $P_{O_2}$ axis) some of the data about impulse traffic in single carotid body afferent fibers from Fig. 4 and data about the ventilatory response to decreased $P_{O_2}$. All three variables are essentially constant at values of $P_{O_2}$ greater than 100 mm Hg. As suggested above, the curve relating impulses/ second in the single afferent fiber from the carotid body is almost an exact mirror image of the Hb-$O_2$ dissociation curve, its slope ever increasing as $P_{O_2}$ falls past 70, 60, 50, and 40 mm Hg. The curve relating ventilation to $P_{O_2}$ (at constant $Pco_2$) is shaped very similarly to the one relating impulse frequency to $P_{O_2}$, showing a perceptible rise at $P_{O_2} = 60$ followed by steeper and steeper rises as the $P_{O_2}$ falls past 50 and 40, and approaching an apparent asymptote at $P_{O_2}$ somewhere in the low 30's. It should be noted that the ventilatory curve

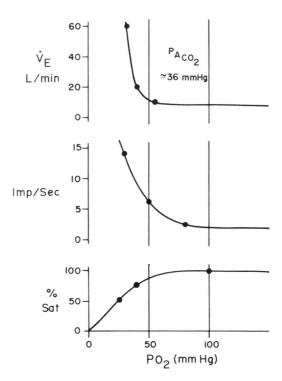

**FIG. 5.** A plot of three different parameters against $P_{O_2}$. From the top down are: Ventilation vs $P_{A_{O_2}}$. (Redrawn from Loeschcke and Gertz, *Pfluegers Arch.*, 267:460, 1958.) Impulses/ second in single carotid body afferent fibers vs $Pa_{O_2}$. (Redrawn from Biscoe, T. J. et al., *J. Physiol. (Lond.)*, 208:121, 1970.) Percentage saturation of Hb in man vs $P_{O_2}$. Note the similar inflection points of the three curves.

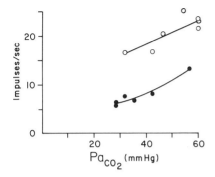

**FIG. 6.** Nerve discharge (impulses/second) recorded from a single chemoreceptor afferent fiber and plotted against $Pa_{CO_2}$. For each curve the pH was kept constant. **Top curve:** pH = 7.25, mean arterial blood pressure = 91 mm Hg; **Bottom curve:** pH = 7.45, mean arterial blood pressure = 85 mm Hg. $Pa_{O_2}$ was 80 mm Hg throughout both curves. (Reproduced with permission from: Biscoe, T. J. et al., The frequency of nerve impulses in single carotid body chemoreceptor afferent fibers recorded *in vivo* with intact circulation. *J. Physiol. (Lond.)*, 208:121, 1970.)

would be much less steep if $P_{CO_2}$ were allowed to change as ventilation tended to increase. $CO_2$ (acting mainly through the central or medullary chemoreceptors) is a far stronger stimulator of ventilation than is hypoxia, and thus a small drop in $P_{CO_2}$ would offset much of the ventilatory stimulation generated by a large decrease in $P_{O_2}$.

But $CO_2$ and $[H^+]$ can also stimulate the carotid body. Figure 6 plots impulses/second recorded from single carotid body afferent nerve fibers as $Pa_{CO_2}$ is raised at each of two constant pH's. Both the lower points ($pH_a = 7.45$) and the upper points ($pH_a = 7.25$) could be fitted very well with straight lines, a very different kind of response curve than the hyperbolic one generated by hypoxia. Although the two curves are roughly parallel, the curve determined at the lower, more acid $pH_a$ is shifted upward toward higher impulse traffic. This demonstrates the specific effect of $[H^+]$ on the carotid body. For example, at a $P_{CO_2}$ of 32 mm Hg, the pH of 7.45 generates about 7 impulses/second, while the pH of 7.25 results in about 17 impulses/second. Of course, the $Pa_{O_2}$ and arterial blood pressure were kept constant throughout the gathering of these data.

## STRUCTURE OF CAROTID BODY

The carotid body is made up of a population of at least two different types of "glomus cells," sympathetic and parasympathetic nerve cells, and afferent neurons. One of the possible models of their functional interactions is shown in Fig. 7. Here, type A glomus cells form reciprocal synapses with each other, with type B cells, and with the glossopharyngeal afferents, while sympathetic and parasympathetic neurons regulate carotid body blood flow.

There is absolutely no agreement among workers in this field about the mechanism(s) by which the changes in $P_{O_2}$, $P_{CO_2}$, and pH bring about impulse traffic in the afferent nerves. McDonald and Mitchell, who have proposed this model, believe that the chemosensitive cells are the afferent nerve endings themselves, rather than one or another of the glomus cells. This idea is supported by the finding that neuromas forming on the cut ends of carotid sinus afferent nerves

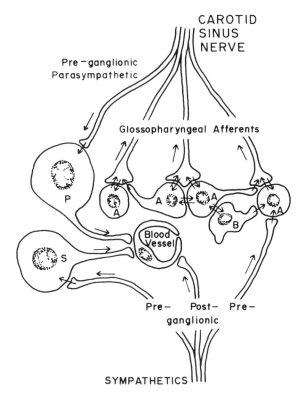

**FIG. 7.** Neural circuit model of the rat carotid body according to McDonald and Mitchell. They postulate that the carotid sinus nerve fibers are chemosensitive whereas glomus cells are dopaminergic inhibitory interneurons. A and B are two subtypes of glomus cells. P and S are parasympathetic and sympathetic ganglion cells, respectively, which regulate carotid body blood flow. *Arrows* indicate direction of nerve fiber activity, and *side-by-side arrows* oriented in opposite directions indicate reciprocal synapses. (Reproduced with permission from: McDonald, D. M. and R. A. Mitchell, The innervation of glomus cells, ganglion cells and blood vessels in the rat carotid body: A quantitative ultrastructural analysis. *J. Neurocytol.,* 4:177, 1975.)

show chemosensitivity without the presence of any glomus cells. These authors believe that the glomus cells, being rich in dopamine, are inhibitory interneurons that modulate the impulse generation by the afferent endings.

The autonomic nervous regulation of blood flow in the carotid body may play an important part in its chemosensitive role. Although it only weighs about 2 mg, the carotid body is believed to have a huge blood flow relative to its weight [as high as 2,000 ml/(100 g tissue·min)], and a very intense metabolic rate as well. Because of the enormous blood supply, there is normally a very small a-v difference for $O_2$ (about 3 ml $O_2$/liter blood), and the tissue $Po_2$ is kept quite near the arterial $Po_2$. Cutting the sympathetics has been shown to increase carotid body blood flow, and stimulating them has been shown to decrease the flow. Thus, an alteration in the sympathetic outflow to the carotid body could change the $Po_2$ to which the chemosensitive cells were exposed, even without the arterial $Po_2$ having changed.

### Central or Medullary Chemoreceptors

That there were some sites in the brain sensitive to elevations of arterial $Pco_2$ and capable of strongly stimulating ventilation in response to those elevations has been known for a long time. It was not until the early 1960's, however, that Mitchell's group localized them precisely to the ventrolateral surface of the medulla oblongata, as seen in Fig. 8. Mitchell's chemosensitive areas (CSA) are bilaterally located at the level of nerve roots 8–11, and are very superficial (no deeper than 0.2 mm). Other superficial areas of chemosensitivity have been identified since then at about the level of the nerve root of cranial nerve 12.

All of these areas have been identified physiologically, but not yet anatomically. That is, we know that the local application of liquids that are acid or in equilibrium with high $Pco_2$ stimulates breathing within seconds; and that substances that depress neural function like cold and local anesthetics quickly depress breathing, but we do not yet know what neural elements are responsible for the chemosensitivity. These areas are insensitive to hypoxia.

Since these receptive areas are so near the surface of the brain, the composition of their extracellular fluid (ECF) is influenced both by the composition of cerebrospinal fluid (CSF) and by that of the blood. CSF is in relatively free communication with the ECF of the chemosensitive elements, the only barriers being a layer of ependymal cells and a more or less tortuous pathway of ECF. These considerations would lead one to expect compositions of CSF and brain ECF to be similar, and current evidence shows this to be true, under nonhypoxic conditions. (When brain cells are hypoxic, they generate relatively large amounts of lactic acid, causing their ECF to be more acid than the CSF.)

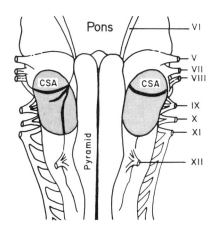

**FIG. 8.** Chemosensitive areas (CSA) on the ventral surface of the medulla. (Reproduced with permission from Mitchell, R. A. and J. W. Severinghaus, Cerebrospinal fluid and regulation of respiration, *Physiol. for Physicians*, 3(3), 1965.)

Normally, the acidity of brain ECF can be changed quickly only through changes in the $P_{CO_2}$ of the blood perfusing the brain, and not at all quickly through changes in blood $[HCO_3^-]$. This selectivity is an expression of the general tightness of the barrier between blood and ECF in brain, fat soluble substances such as gases and anesthetics moving quite freely while ions are greatly restricted. Figure 9 is a hypothetical model of the medullary chemoreceptors embodying some of these particulars. It shows the chemosensitive cell and its ECF being exposed to the composition of CSF sperficially and to the composition of blood more deeply. It shows that $CO_2$ is freely diffusible throughout the system; $H^+$ and $HCO_3^-$ can exchange relatively freely between ECF and CSF, but their movement is severely restricted between blood and ECF. A rise in blood $P_{CO_2}$ will raise $P_{CO_2}$ in the brain causing $CO_2$ to hydrate there forming $H_2CO_3$, which will dissociate as usual forming $H^+$ and $HCO_3^-$. Thus, raising blood $P_{CO_2}$ can acidify the ECF in the vicinity of the chemoreceptive cells, leading to a stimulation of ventilation.

This stimulation, while it begins within seconds of the elevation in arterial $P_{CO_2}$, takes minutes before reaching a new steady state (assuming that the elevated arterial $P_{CO_2}$ is maintained). The reader will remember that the carotid bodies' response time was much shorter, a change in arterial $P_{O_2}$ or $P_{CO_2}$ causing a change in impulse frequency which began as soon as the blood reached it and very rapidly reached a steady level. The response of the carotid bodies can be so prompt because their enormous blood flow [2,000 ml/(100 g/min)] causes their tissue to reach equilibrium with new levels of blood $P_{O_2}$ and $P_{CO_2}$ almost instantly.

The blood flow to the brain is only about 45 ml/(100 g/min). Thus, while a change in arterial $P_{CO_2}$ *begins* to change brain $P_{CO_2}$ very quickly, it takes perhaps 5–10 minutes before the brain $P_{CO_2}$ (and the pH of its ECF) stabilizes at a new level.

What about $[HCO_3^-]$ of CSF and brain ECF? We already know that a rise in blood $P_{CO_2}$ will cause the blood $[HCO_3^-]$ to rise, the amount of change being dependent on the concentration of protein buffers in the blood. The rise in blood $[HCO_3^-]$ would tend to favor the diffusion of $HCO_3^-$ from blood to

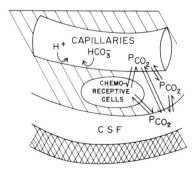

**FIG. 9.** The chemosensitive cells are influenced by the compositions of both blood and CSF. The barriers between blood and brain are such that ions pass with difficulty while lipid-soluble molecules (anesthetics, respiratory gases) pass easily. Thus, the acid–base status of the chemoreceptive cells can be changed quickly only through changing arterial $P_{CO_2}$. Changing arterial $[HCO_3^-]$ or $[H^+]$ does not lead to quick changes in these parameters in brain cells in general or in chemóreceptive cells in particular.

CSF, but the "tightness" of the blood-brain barrier makes this movement very slow. The CSF formed actively at the choroid plexures may also have a higher $[HCO_3^-]$ under these conditions. The raising of the $P_{CO_2}$ in CSF and brain ECF will cause the hydration of $CO_2$ to $H_2CO_3$ and its subsequent dissociation to $H^+$ and $HCO_3^-$ in those fluids. Since there are essentially no protein buffers in either fluid, however, the amount of $HCO_3^-$ formed by this means is immeasurably small.

Finally, the increased $P_{CO_2}$ will tend to cause hydration of $CO_2$ in brain cells and subsequent formation of $HCO_3^-$ by dissociation of $H_2CO_3$. The amount of $HCO_3^-$ formed by this means can be quite large, since there is plenty of intracellular protein to buffer the $H^+$ formed and thus prevent the reactions from reaching a new equilibrium until lots of $HCO_3^-$ have been formed (there is also lots of carbonic anhydrase intracellularly, so the hydration happens very quickly). This extra $HCO_3^-$ can then leak out of the cells into the CSF and brain ECF to raise their $[HCO_3^-]$, but the process occurs fairly slowly due to the low anion permeability of brain cells. (This whole sequence of events occurs within a fraction of a second in red cells as they pass through the tissues and pick up $CO_2$ because their anion permeability is huge!)

The result of all of these processes, and perhaps many others, is that $[HCO_3^-]$ of the CSF and brain ECF begins to rise soon after a step rise in blood $P_{CO_2}$. It reaches a new steady level some 8 hours to a day after the rise was initiated, at which time the CSF and brain ECF pH have almost returned to normal. Thus, the medullary chemoreceptors are initially made quite acid by a sizeable rise in $P_{CO_2}$. If the elevated level of $P_{CO_2}$ is maintained, however, the rise in $[HCO_3^-]$ of brain fluids returns the pH of those fluids back toward normal in a day or so, minimizing the excess ventilatory stimulation generated by the medullary chemoreceptors even though the $P_{CO_2}$ remains high.

## INTERACTION OF PERIPHERAL AND MEDULLARY CHEMORECEPTORS—HYPERCAPNIA

Raising the arterial $P_{CO_2}$ provides a very strong chemical stimulus to breathing, a rise of only 2 mm Hg capable of doubling resting ventilation in some subjects. One of the reasons that a rise in $P_{CO_2}$ is such a potent drive to breathing is that, unlike changes in $P_{O_2}$ and pH, it acts on both the peripheral and medullary chemoreceptors in the same direction (to increase ventilation). Because of this exquisite sensitivity, our resting breathing waxes and wanes as $P_{CO_2}$ tends to change, managing to keep alveolar and arterial $P_{CO_2}$ remarkably constant at sea level.

### Acute Changes in $P_{CO_2}$

The $CO_2$ response curve has often been used to quantitate the "sensitivity" of the breathing control system to acute increases in $P_{CO_2}$. In the commonly used steady-state method, ventilation and $P_{CO_2}$ (usually end-tidal) are measured at the end of each of a series of 10-minute time periods. The inspired $P_{CO_2}$ may be zero in the first time period, then be held constant at 20 mm Hg for the next time period, then at 30 mm Hg for the next, perhaps reaching a high of 35 mm Hg during the fourth period. The inspired $P_{CO_2}$ is then dropped for the fifth period, more during the sixth, and may again be zero during the seventh.

If the breathing were to remain unchanged during these changes in inspired $P_{CO_2}$, then the alveolar $P_{CO_2}$ would be expected to rise just as much as the inspired, in each new steady state. Of course, the elevated alveolar and arterial $P_{CO_2}$ actually causes the ventilation to increase, and the amount of the increase in alveolar and arterial $P_{CO_2}$ for any given rise in inspired $P_{CO_2}$ depends on the vigor of the ventilatory response. Back a few chapters we developed the equation $P_{A_{CO_2}} = 863$ mm Hg ($\dot{V}_{CO_2}$, STPD)/$\dot{V}_A$, BTPS) to quantitate the steady-state relationship among these three variables. In the development of this equation, we assumed that the inspired $P_{CO_2}$ was zero, as it is in normal situations. Under conditions in which the inspired $P_{CO_2}$ may get significantly greater than zero, the following form of that equation is a good approximation to the truth: $P_{A_{CO_2}} - P_{I_{CO_2}} = 863$ mm Hg ($\dot{V}_{CO_2}$, STPD)/$\dot{V}_A$, BTPS). In other words, it is the difference between inspired and alveolar $P_{CO_2}$ that depends on the ratio of $CO_2$ production to alveolar ventilation. During the steady states of a resting $CO_2$ response curve, $\dot{V}_{CO_2}$ will remain approximately constant. Therefore, during the determination of that curve, the difference between alveolar and inspired $P_{CO_2}$ varies only as $1/\dot{V}_A$.

Suppose, for example, a subject's $P_{A_{CO_2}} = 40$ mm Hg and his $\dot{V}_A = 5$ liters/min during the first 10-minute period of a $CO_2$ response curve (while $P_{I_{CO_2}} = 0$). His $P_{A_{CO_2}} - P_{I_{CO_2}}$ thus is 40 mm Hg. Suppose, in a later 10-minute steady state, his $P_{A_{CO_2}}$ is now 43 mm Hg as a result of his $P_{I_{CO_2}}$ being raised to 30 mm Hg. What is his $\dot{V}_A$ in this new steady state? Well, the difference between his $P_{A_{CO_2}}$ and $P_{I_{CO_2}}$ is now 13 mm Hg, about one-third what it was in the first period. Therefore, his $\dot{V}_A$ must be three times what it was then, or about 15 liters/min.

Figure 10 shows data plotted from a $CO_2$ response curve determined on a 29-year-old healthy male. $P_{A_{O_2}}$ was kept at 200 mm Hg throughout so as to avoid any variable hypoxic stimulation of breathing. The seven steady-state points have been plotted, and a straight line of best fit, calculated by the method of least squares, has been superimposed on the graph. This response can be characterized by the position and slope of that calculated line. In this case, the X-intercept (where ventilation would be zero) is 38.83 mm Hg, and the slope is 3.24 (liters/min)/mm Hg. In general, these normoxic or slightly hyperoxic $CO_2$ response curves in normal, sea-level men will have X-intercepts between 35 and 40 mm Hg and slopes which vary between 1 and 4 (liters/min)/mm Hg.

Because this steady-state measurement of ventilatory response to $CO_2$ is time

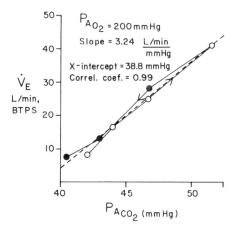

FIG. 10. A graph of ventilatory response to inhaled $CO_2$, sometimes called a "$CO_2$ response curve." While the $P_{A_{O_2}}$ is kept at 200 mm Hg through enrichment of the inspired gas with $O_2$, the inspired $P_{CO_2}$ is raised in a series of steps to raise the $P_{A_{CO_2}}$ and $\dot{V}_E$ in a series of steps. At each step, the inspired $P_{CO_2}$ is kept steady for 10 minutes, during the last 3 of which $P_{A_{CO_2}}$ and $\dot{V}_E$ are measured.

consuming and fairly unpleasant (it is uncomfortable to breathe mixtures of gas high in $CO_2$ for any length of time), alternative methods have been explored. One of these which is popular now is the rebreathing technique developed by Read in the late 1960's. After a period of quiet resting breathing to and from room air, the subject is connected to a bag containing about 7% $CO_2$ and 93% $O_2$ and asked to take a few deep breaths. This quickly results in equality of $P_{CO_2}$ among the bag, the subject's lungs, and his arterial and mixed venous blood if the bag is of appropriate size (subject's vital capacity + about 1 liter). Thereafter, $P_{CO_2}$ rises linearly by about 6 mm Hg/min for the balance of the determination, which only lasts for 3–4 minutes. The $CO_2$ response curve can then be constructed using values of ventilation for each of a series of half-minute periods along with the $P_{CO_2}$ at the midpoint of each period. This method tends to result in slopes similar to the steady-state method, but positions displaced to the right of the steady-state method by 6–8 mm Hg.

### Chronic Changes in $P_{CO_2}$—Acclimatization to High $P_{CO_2}$

It has been pointed out in this chapter that increases in $P_{CO_2}$, if maintained, cause increases in brain $[HCO_3^-]$ which level off in a day or so. The converse is also true; that is, decreases in $P_{CO_2}$ lead chronically to decreases in brain $[HCO_3^-]$ with about the same time course. What these changes in brain $[HCO_3^-]$ do is to "reset" the response range of the medullary chemoreceptors! Let me illustrate with an example. Suppose an animal's control $Pa_{CO_2}$ is 40 mm Hg and his $pH_a$ is 7.40, giving a $[HCO_3^-]_a$ of 23.9 mEq/liter. Under these control circumstances his CSF $P_{CO_2}$ is 50.8 and his CSF pH is 7.314, giving a CSF [$HCO_3^-$] of 24.1 mEq/liter. The animal is now exposed to an elevated $P_{I_{CO_2}}$ so as to raise his $P_{A_{CO_2}}$ to 55 mm Hg and keep it there for 6 hours. One can calculate (from the measured CSF $P_{CO_2}$ of 68 mm Hg and assuming no change in CSF [$HCO_3^-$]) that the brain ECF (BECF) pH would acutely be very low, about 7.17, and would stimulate the medullary chemoreceptors greatly. Some 6 hours later, as a result of processes that have been mentioned in this chapter, his CSF [$HCO_3^-$] will have risen to 29 mEq/liter, thus raising the pH of the BECF to 7.25, a much less vigorous ventilatory stimulant to the medullary chemoreceptors. To lower the pH acutely to 7.17 would require raising the arterial $P_{CO_2}$ to 70 mm Hg at this brain ECF [$HCO_3^-$]. Acutely lowering the arterial $P_{CO_2}$ to the control value of 40 mm Hg would cause a brain ECF pH of about 7.38 at this level of brain ECF [$HCO_3^-$], a pH that would remove any drive to breathing from the medullary chemoreceptors.

Thus, chronic exposure to high $P_{CO_2}$ has reset the medullary chemoreceptors toward higher $P_{CO_2}$ by raising the brain ECF [$HCO_3^-$]. Said another way, the higher brain ECF [$HCO_3^-$] makes any given arterial $P_{CO_2}$ translate into a higher and less stimulatory brain ECF pH than it did at the lower brain ECF [$HCO_3^-$]. One would predict from these considerations that a $CO_2$ response curve measured after the chronic exposure would be shifted toward higher $P_{CO_2}$ from the control curve, and this prediction is borne out experimentally. The process has been called "acclimatization to high $P_{CO_2}$."

This resetting of the medullary chemoreceptors upon chronic exposures to high arterial $P_{CO_2}$ has important clinical relevance. Many a patient with one or another form of respiratory insufficiency does retain $CO_2$ chronically, becoming acclimatized to the high $P_{CO_2}$. An acute respiratory infection can greatly worsen the respiratory insufficiency so that the patient finds it necessary to visit a hospital—dyspneic, cyanotic, confused, and alarmed. $P_{a_{CO_2}}$ can be alarmingly high and $O_2$ saturation astonishingly low upon admission, but the arterial pH is usually fairly well compensated, being in the neighborhood of 7.3. For example, a series of 16 emphysematous patients in the throes of such emergency admissions to an English hospital had $P_{a_{CO_2}}$ of 52–86 mm Hg, arterial $O_2$ saturations of 36–81%, while their $pH_a$ ranged from 7.2 to 7.39. Their arterial $P_{O_2}$ (calculated by me from the percentage of saturation and the arterial pH) ranged between 26 and 51 mm Hg, the average being 37 mm Hg.

Clearly, in some of these patients, the arterial $O_2$ saturation is low enough to be life-threatening, and in all of them the arterial $P_{O_2}$ is low enough to be providing most of the drive to whatever level of breathing they are managing. The $P_{a_{CO_2}}$, while very high, is providing very little drive to breathing because these patients are acclimatized to it.

These patients needed supplemental $O_2$ and were given it in $O_2$ tents with inspired gas mixtures estimated at 40–50% $O_2$, raising their arterial $O_2$ saturations to 86–100%. The next few days saw their $P_{a_{CO_2}}$ rise as high as 187 mm Hg, their $pH_a$ fall as low as 6.83, and stupor and coma to be the rule! Six of this series of patients died, partially or largely as a result of this fulminating respiratory acidosis.

## CO₂ NARCOSIS

The problem seems to be that $CO_2$, while stimulatory to breathing at normal levels, becomes an anesthetic when its partial pressure rises high enough. Any of these patients whose $Pa_{CO_2}$ rose above 100 mm Hg showed disturbances of mental state, and any whose $Pa_{CO_2}$ rose above 120 mm Hg were comatose. So the supplemental $O_2$, while it relieved their cyanosis, also removed much of their drive to breathe, allowing $CO_2$ to accumulate to narcotic levels. Of course, as the $CO_2$ level rises into the narcotic range, the drive to breathe decreases further and further, a classic positive-feedback system!

This study and many others have led to caution in the administration of $O_2$ to patients with chronic $CO_2$ retention. Oxygen must be given to some of these patients, but only enough to relieve life-threatening hypoxia. The arterial $Po_2$ must be left low enough to provide a strong drive to breathing via the carotid bodies. Artificial ventilation also may play a part in the current therapy of these patients.

## ACCLIMATIZATION TO LOW $Pco_2$

From what has been said already, it should be obvious that the chronic maintenance of a lower than normal $Pco_2$ will lead to acclimatization to that lower $Pco_2$. The brain ECF $[HCO_3^-]$ decreases, causing any given brain $Pco_2$ to make the environment around the medullary chemoreceptors more acid than it normally would be at that $Pco_2$. Thus, ventilation will be driven more strongly than usual at any given $Pco_2$, and the $CO_2$ response curve will be shifted toward lower $Pco_2$. Because cerebral blood flow decreases as the $Pco_2$ decreases, the brain may be made somewhat hypoxic at $Pco_2$ less than about 20 mm Hg even if the arterial blood $Po_2$ is normal or above normal. This brain tissue hypoxia will increase lactic acid production by the brain, thus leading to even more profound lowering of the brain ECF $[HCO_3^-]$ than one might expect from the lowering of the $Pco_2$ alone. The evolutionary pressures, which have retained this tendency toward lactic acidosis in the brain when $Pco_2$ is dropped greatly, probably involve homeostatis of brain pH. The lactic acidosis prevents the brain from getting as alkalotic as it otherwise would.

## INTERACTION OF PERIPHERAL AND MEDULLARY CHEMORECEPTORS—HYPOXIA

Hypoxia (if sufficiently severe) acts through the peripheral chemoreceptors to cause an immediate increase in ventilation which lowers $Pco_2$ and raises pH as usual. This initial increase in ventilation is rather small. For instance, breathing 12% $O_2$ at sea level or normal air at 13,500 ft. might lead acutely to an increase of 10% or less. The main reason ventilation changes so little under these conditions is that the peripheral and medullary chemoreceptors work against one another. The hypoxia, working through the peripheral chemoreceptors, tends to increase ventilation. As ventilation increases, however, the decrease in $P_{CO_2}$ inhibits the medullary chemoreceptors (and, to a much lesser extent, the decrease in $P_{CO_2}$ and the increase in pH reduce the carotid chemoreceptors's drive to breathing). Since ventilation is so exquisitely sensitive to changes in $P_{CO_2}$, a small decrease in $P_{CO_2}$ (caused by only a small increase in ventilation) suffices to offset much of the ventilatory stimulation which the hypoxia might otherwise cause. All of these changes are completely reversible during the first few minutes of hypoxia. Returning the inspired $P_{O_2}$ to normal, promptly returns the ventilation, blood $P_{O_2}$, $P_{CO_2}$, and pH back to normal.

Figure 11 shows the $P_{A_{CO_2}}$ and expired ventilation ($\dot{V}_E$) of a healthy subject before, during, and after 8 hours of hypoxia ($P_{A_{O_2}}$ of 45–50 mm Hg). The normoxic (before) values of $P_{A_{CO_2}}$ and $\dot{V}_E$, respectively, were 38.2 mm Hg and 6.5 liters/min. Hypoxia raised $\dot{V}_E$ immediately to about 8.6 liters/min and lowered $P_{A_{CO_2}}$ immediately to 35.9 mm Hg.

## VENTILATORY ACCLIMATIZATION TO CHRONIC HYPOXIA

Figure 11 also shows that, if the hypoxia is prolonged beyond a few minutes, the ventilation continues to increase, and the $P_{A_{CO_2}}$ continues to decrease, the levels of both tending to plateau by 8 hours or so. These chronic levels of $P_{A_{CO_2}}$ (29.7 mm Hg) and $\dot{V}_E$ (10.9 liters/min) are changed greatly from the normoxic ones. Figure 11 further demonstrates that the changes are persistent; removing the hypoxia after a chronic exposure now only brings $P_{A_{CO_2}}$ and $\dot{V}_E$ part way back to their prehypoxic levels. It will take many hours to a few days of chronic normoxia before this state of Ventilatory Acclimatization to Chronic Hypoxia has completely disappeared. The ventilatory acclimatization in studies such as these may be measured by the difference between $CO_2$ response curves determined before the chronic exposure and those determined immediately afterwards, both times with sufficient $O_2$ added to eliminate the effects of hypoxia during the curves. Figure 12 shows such a pair of $CO_2$ response curves obtained before and after an 8-hour exposure to hypoxia ($P_{A_{O_2}} = 49$ mm Hg) and low $P_{CO_2}$ ($P_{A_{CO_2}} = 30$ mm Hg). The $CO_2$ response curve determined after the exposure is shifted considerably to the left of the control curve (toward lower $P_{A_{CO_2}}$) and is steeper than the control curve. Any given $P_{A_{CO_2}}$ after the exposure causes a much higher ventilation than it did before. For example, the resting $P_{A_{CO_2}}$ of about 41.3 mm Hg drives breathing up to nearly 40 liters/min after the exposure compared with about 8 liters/min before it.

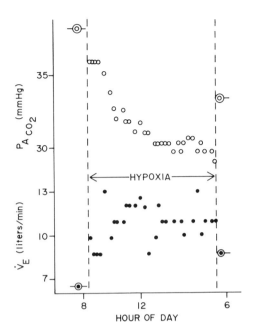

**FIG. 11.** The time course of $P_{A_{CO_2}}$ and $\dot{V}_E$ before, during, and after an 8-hour hypoxic exposure in a normal male. The ventilation increases immediately and causes the $P_{A_{CO_2}}$ to decrease immediately upon the initiation of hypoxia. These parameters continue to change during the 8 hours, the $\dot{V}_E$ finally leveling off at about 11 liters/min and the $P_{A_{CO_2}}$ leveling off at about 30 mm Hg. Upon relieving the hypoxia, $\dot{V}_E$ quickly falls part way, and $P_{A_{CO_2}}$ quickly rises part way back toward the control values. Thus, a persistent change in these parameters has been brought about by the chronic hypoxia.

## HOW DOES VENTILATORY ACCLIMATIZATION TO CHRONIC HYPOXIA HELP THE ORGANISM?

Very simply—this process minimizes the $O_2$ desaturation of arterial blood. Let us consider an example of an exposure to a moderately high altitude in each of two individuals: One who undergoes ventilatory acclimatization, and one who does not. The individuals will be identical in other respects.

Table 1 compares the values one might find in two sea-level natives, both of whom had ascended to an altitude of 14,000 ft. 3 days ago, but only one of whom underwent ventilatory acclimatization to the chronic hypoxia. The inspired $P_{O_2}$ is 84 mm Hg for both, since $P_B$ at that altitude is about 447 mm Hg. The acclimatized individual's $\dot{V}_E$ is up at 10 liters/min, while the nonacclimatized individual's $\dot{V}_E$ is at 7 liters/min, representing $\dot{V}_A$'s of 7.5 and 5 liters/min, respectively. These values of $\dot{V}_A$ will result in $P_{A_{CO_2}}$ of 26 and 40 mm Hg, respectively. Plugging these values into the alveolar gas equation with $R = 0.8$ gives $P_{A_{O_2}}$'s of 53 and 36 mm Hg, respectively, which convert

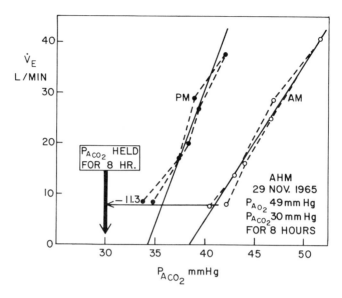

**FIG. 12.** $CO_2$ response curves measured before and after the subject's exposure to 8 hour of hypoxia ($P_{A_{O_2}}$ = 49 mm Hg) and hypocapnia ($P_{A_{CO_2}}$ = 30 mm Hg). The "after" curve is shifted to the left and increased in steepness. ($P_{A_{O_2}}$ was kept at 200 mm Hg during the measurement of both curves.) Thus, a persistent change in the subject's ventilatory response to $CO_2$ has been brought about by the chronic hypoxia and hypocapnia.

to 48 and 31 mm Hg when the A-a gradient of 5 mm Hg is considered. These values of $Pa_{O_2}$ will result in $O_2$ saturations of 84 and 59%, respectively, a huge difference from the functional standpoint.

A sea-level native whose $Pa_{O_2}$ is 48 mm Hg and whose arterial $O_2$ saturation is 84% after 3 days of altitude residence may feel irritable and short of breath, but will be alert, reasoning, and capable of performing most physical tasks that were possible for him to perform at sea level. The sea-level native whose breathing did not change at all upon the chronic hypoxic exposure will have

TABLE 1. *Effect of acclimatization to altitude on $P_{A_{O_2}}$*

|  | $P_{I_{O_2}}$ (mm Hg) | $\dot{V}_E$ (liters/min) | $P_{A_{CO_2}}$ (mm Hg) | $Pa_{O_2}$ (mm Hg) | % Sat. of Hb | Functional state |
|---|---|---|---|---|---|---|
| Normally acclimatizing subject | 84 | 10 | 26 | 48 | 84 | Alert and physically able |
| Nonacclimatizing subject | 84 | 7 | 40 | 31 | 59 | Stuporous or comatose |

Three days after ascent to 14,000 ft. R.Q. assumed to be 0.8, A-a gradient for $P_{O_2}$ assumed to be 5 mm Hg at altitude, $\dot{V}_E$ of 10 liters/min associated with $\dot{V}_A$ of 7.5 liters/min, and $\dot{V}_E$ of 7 liters/min associated with $\dot{V}_A$ of 5 liters/min. $P_B$ = 447 mm Hg.

a normal $PA_{CO_2}$ of 40 mm Hg leading to a $Pa_{O_2}$ of 31 and arterial $O_2$ saturation of 59%. He would do better to stay at sea level! These levels of oxygenation will leave him stuporous at best and comatose at worst, and unable to care for himself in either event.

## MECHANISMS OF VENTILATORY ACCLIMATIZATION TO CHRONIC HYPOXIA

It is well established that the initial rapid hyperventilation occurring within seconds of onset of hypoxic exposure is mediated by the carotid bodies. Unfortunately, the mechanisms responsible for the second, slower ventilatory change, which occurs over the next day or so of hypoxic exposure, are incompletely understood. Certainly the CSF $[HCO_3^-]$ decreases with about the same time course as the breathing change; however, the $P_{CO_2}$ in the brain is also decreasing rapidly, and the two changing variables result in a quite alkaline CSF when the breathing has reached its highest level. If CSF composition always gave us a good idea of the composition of brain ECF (and in particular, the composition of the brain ECF in the vicinity of the medullary chemoreceptors), we would be forced to conclude that something unrelated to brain pH was driving breathing at this time. The arterial blood is still quite alkaline at this point, and its $P_{CO_2}$ and $P_{O_2}$ are less stimulatory to the carotid bodies than they were upon the initiation of the hypoxia. If the ECF in the neighborhood of the medullary chemoreceptors were also less stimulatory (more alkaline) than it was upon the initial hypoxic exposure, some factors unrelated to the usual chemical stimuli acting through these chemoreceptors would have to be invoked to explain why the ventilation is so high chronically.

Investigators have invoked other factors in the face of this apparent impasse, but it may not be necessary to do so. Recent evidence strengthens the feeling of many workers in this field that CSF composition may be quite different from brain ECF composition during hypoxia. That is, the greatly increased lactic acid production by the brain during hypoxia may serve to acidify the brain interstitial and intracellular fluid far more than the CSF. Thus, although the CSF pH may be quite alkaline at the height of the ventilatory increase, the environment of the medullary chemoreceptors may be sufficiently acidified to explain the increased drive to breathing.

### REFERENCES

1. Berger, A. J., Mitchell, R. A., and Severinghaus, J. W. (1977): Regulation of respiration. *N. Engl. J. Med.*, 297:92–97, 138–143, 194–201.
2. Biscoe, T. J., Purves, M. J., and Sampson, S. R. (1970): The frequency of nerve impulses in single carotid body chemoreceptor fibres recorded in *in vivo* with intact circulation. *J. Physiol. (Lond.)*, 208:121–131.
3. Mitchell, R. A., and Berger, A. J. (1975): Neural control of respiration. *Am. Rev. Respir. Dis.*, 111:206.

4. Mitchell, R. A., Loeschcke, H. H., Massion, W. H., and Severinghaus, J. W. (1963): Respiratory responses mediated through superficial chemosensitive areas on the medulla. *J. Appl. Physiol.,* 18:523–533.
5. Westlake, E. K., Simpson, T., and Kaye, M. (1955): Carbon dioxide narcosis in emphysema. *Q. J. Med.,* 24:155–173.

## PROBLEMS

1. The graph in Fig. 13 shows a line obtained by increasing $P_{A_{CO_2}}$ by adding $CO_2$ to the inspired air while keep $P_{A_{O_2}}$ constant at 100 mm Hg in a single subject. Which of the following statements provides the best description of points *a–e* plotted on the graph by manipulation performed on the same subject:

   A. Subject at rest is breathing a gas mixture enriched with $CO_2$ and $O_2$.
   B. Subject at rest breathing normal air at sea level.
   C. Subject at rest breathing normal air at high altitude (about 12,000 ft.).
   D. Subject is asphyxic.
   E. Toward the end of 30 seconds of voluntary hyperventilation.

2. The medullary chemoreceptors

   a. respond quickly to changes in arterial acidity at constant $P_{A_{CO_2}}$
   b. arc primarily sensitive to changes in brain $P_{O_2}$
   c. are inhibited by increases in brain extracellular fluid acidity
   d. can be physiologically stimulated quickly only through changes in $P_{A_{CO_2}}$
   e. are probably located deep within the medulla but have not been anatomically located as yet

3. Hypoxia influences respiration quickly only through its stimulatory effect

   a. directly on the respiratory centers
   b. directly on the lungs
   c. on the medullary chemoreceptors

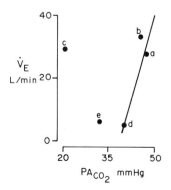

**FIG. 13.** A graph of $\dot{V}_E$ in liters/min vs $P_{A_{CO_2}}$ in mm Hg. The line shows the normal response when the $P_{A_{O_2}}$ is kept at 100 mm Hg and the steady state is allowed to develop at each level of inspired $P_{CO_2}$.

d. on the carotid and aortic chemoreceptors
e. directly on the Hb-$O_2$ dissociation curve

4. A lightly anesthetized patient is still capable of spontaneous breathing and is artificially ventilated at his normal tidal volume, but at twice his normal frequency, with a gas mixture of 50% $O_2$ and 50% $N_2$ for 10 minutes. On cessation of this artificial ventilation, the patient fails to breathe for 1 minute. Probably the most important cause of this temporary apnea is decreased activity of the

   a. peripheral chemoreceptors because of the high $P_{O_2}$
   b. peripheral chemoreceptors because of the low $P_{CO_2}$
   c. PSRs that inhibit inspiration
   d. medullary chemoreceptors because of low $P_{CO_2}$
   e. medullary chemoreceptors because of the high $P_{O_2}$

5. Transection of the brainstem in the mid pons results in

   a. apneustic respiration
   b. loss of rhythmic respiratory efforts
   c. very slow, very deep breathing
   d. loss of respiratory response to elevated $P_{ACO_2}$
   e. increase in respiratory frequency
   f. slight slowing and slight deepening of breathing

6. An acute exposure for 10 minutes to hypoxia ($P_{AO_2} = 50$ mm Hg) would, in a normal subject, cause

   a. an increase in arterial $P_{CO_2}$
   b. a decrease in arterial pH
   c. a decrease in activity of the medullary chemoreceptors
   d. a decrease in activity of the peripheral chemoreceptors
   e. a decrease in the pH of CSF

## ANSWERS

1. **A:** Since the line depicts the $CO_2$ response curve of this person while his $P_{AO_2}$ is kept at 100 mm Hg, and our subject has elevated $P_{CO_2}$ and hyperoxia, his ventilation will be slightly less than the line would lead us to expect at any given $P_{ACO_2}$. This will happen because the carotid chemoreceptors, while they drive breathing very little at $P_{AO_2} = 100$ mm Hg, do contribute some drive to breathing. This drive is lessened when $P_{O_2}$ is raised. Answer is (a).
**B:** This person would be expected to have a normal $P_{ACO_2}$ (of 40 mm Hg, if male) and to lie on the bottom end of the $CO_2$ response line, since $P_{AO_2}$

at sea level while breathing normal air *will* be about 100 mm Hg. Answer is (d).

**C:** This subject will be hyperventilating due to the hypoxic stimulus of the altitude, and his ventilation will therefore be increased, which will have reduced his $P_{A_{CO_2}}$. Point (e) has ventilation increased by six-fifths over the control and $P_{A_{CO_2}}$ decreased to about five-sixths of the control, and is therefore the answer.

**D:** Asphyxia means that both hypoxia and elevated $P_{CO_2}$ are present. Point (b) is at $P_{A_{CO_2}}$ of about 45.5, but the ventilation is greater than the line indicates it ought to be at a normal $P_{A_{O_2}}$ of 100 mm Hg. Thus, something else is driving the person's breathing, like hypoxia.

**E:** Voluntary hyperventilation will drive down $P_{A_{CO_2}}$ and, in the new steady state, $P_{A_{CO_2}}$ will have decreased by the reciprocal of the factor by which ventilation has increased. Thirty seconds, however, will not be nearly enough time for a new steady state to have developed. Thus, point (c), whose ventilation is increased by almost a factor of six, has a $P_{A_{CO_2}}$ that is decreased only to about one-half of the control, but is the answer. Given time, the steady state $P_{A_{CO_2}}$ would decrease all the way down to about 7 mm Hg, if the ventilation were maintained.

2. Answer (d) is the only correct one. Answers (a) and (b) are wrong, (c) is in the wrong direction, and the first phrase in answer (e) is opposite to the truth.

3. Answer (d) is correct.

4. Since $P_{O_2}$ provides little of the resting, sea-level drive to breathing, the apnea cannot be due to elevation of the $P_{O_2}$ above the normal levels. $CO_2$ is the strongest drive to breathing around the normal levels, and $CO_2$ acts primarily through the medullary chemoreceptors. Thus, the important factor must be that the hyperventilation has lowered $P_{CO_2}$ greatly, and the $CO_2$ production of the body takes 1 minute in this subject to bring the $P_{CO_2}$ back up to stimulatory levels. Answer must be (d).

5. Transection of the brainstem in the midpons will remove the influence of the higher, cognitive centers and the pneumotaxic center. The higher centers play little part in automatic control of breathing, but the pneumotaxic center is involved in terminating each inspiration, along with the PSR acting through the Hering-Breuer stretch reflex. Thus, each inspiration will last somewhat longer and be somewhat deeper, and the answer is (f).

6. A $P_{A_{O_2}}$ of 50 mm Hg is low enough to cause some hyperventilation, lowering of $P_{CO_2}$, and raising of pH throughout the body of a normal individual. This rules out alternatives (a), (b), and (e) immediately. An alkalinization

of the brain will certainly decrease the activity of the medullary chemorecep-tors, so alternative (c) is certainly correct. But, doesn't lowering of $P_{CO_2}$ and raising of pH also decrease the activity of the peripheral chemoreceptors, making alternative (d) also correct? It does, of course, but we've got the tail wagging the dog now. The reason for the hyperventilation is hypoxic *stimulation* of the peripheral chemoreceptors, and their activity is thus *up*, making the answer only (c).

# Subject Index

# Subject Index

AF